DO YOU KNOW . . .

- How to spot the warning signs of a second stroke?

- Where to get a restraint-free, state-of-the-art ambulation device—that Medicare will pay for?

- How a "progress diary" will let you see the steps toward recovery?

- Why stroke survivors may spontaneously burst into laughter or crying?

- How a word or picture board can stimulate speech and language?

- What professional techniques will make dressing and undressing easier?

- How to evaluate your own emotional state as a caregiver?

- What to do if you, the caregiver, get depressed or overstressed?

WHEN SOMEONE YOU LOVE HAS A STROKE

Dell Caregiving Guides

The Dell Caregiving Guides

When Someone You Love Has a Stroke

A National Stroke Association Book

Marilynn Larkin

Foreword by Fletcher H. McDowell, M.D.

PRODUCED BY LYNN SONBERG BOOK ASSOCIATES

Published by
Dell Publishing
a division of
Bantam Doubleday Dell Publishing Group, Inc.
1540 Broadway
New York, New York 10036

Research about stroke recovery is ongoing and subject to interpretation. Although every effort has been made to include the most up-to-date and accurate information in this book, there can be no guarantee that what we know about this complex subject won't change with time. The reader should bear in mind that this book should not be used for self-diagnosis or self-treatment, and should consult appropriate medical professionals regarding all health issues.

ISBN: 0-440-21666-4

Published by arrangement with Lynn Sonberg Book Associates, 260 West 72nd Street, Suite 6-C, New York, New York 10023.

Printed in the United States of America

Published simultaneously in Canada

October 1995

10 9 8 7 6 5 4 3

OPM

Contents

Foreword

Stroke happens in a moment but changes lives forever. The very suddenness with which stroke strikes—often without warning—leaves the stroke survivor and family precious little time to prepare for, come to terms with, and adjust to the changes stroke imposes. This makes the first days, weeks, and months a particularly difficult time for the stroke survivor, caregiver, and family.

Stroke affects not only the stroke survivor but the entire family as well. Therefore this book is written for you—the families, the caregivers, and the stroke survivors. National Stroke Association is pleased to present this book to all who find themselves confronting the many challenges stroke creates. For more than ten years National Stroke Association has been working, communicating, and sharing with a great number of our nation's three million stroke survivors and their families.

Our purpose in developing this guide is to share what we have learned from those coping with and overcoming the immediate and lifelong challenges of recovery after stroke. These insights come primarily from stroke survivors and caregivers themselves, but also include the latest important medical information from leading authorities in stroke treatment and rehabilitation.

Recovery from the effects of stroke requires teamwork, and research shows that stroke survivors who have committed caregivers and families improve faster and compensate for their deficits better than do stroke survivors without the immediate caring of others. Therefore the role that caregivers and families play in supporting stroke survivors as they strive to reestablish productive and worthwhile lives cannot be overstated. We hope this book offers helpful guidance and inspiration as you travel forward together toward a meaningful and fulfilling life after stroke. Remember, you are not alone. There are more than three million stroke survivors and their caregivers and families who share similar frustrations, courage, and accomplishments. National Stroke Association stands by you and is here for you as well. Do not hesitate to call upon us.

Fletcher H. McDowell, M.D.
President
National Stroke Association

Acknowledgments

The author wishes to express her deep appreciation to Gary Houser, Vice President; Thelma Edwards, R.N.; and the rest of the staff of the National Stroke Association for their invaluable help and support in this project. She also thanks Ruth Kamerman from OPUS in Hartsdale, New York, and the many stroke survivors and caregivers in that group who shared their stories with her.

Special thanks to Deborah Mitchell for her assistance in preparing the manuscript.

Introduction

Caring for a close family member or friend who has experienced a stroke requires courage, fortitude, and understanding. Now that you have been through the first few days or weeks of fear and worry, the challenges of assisting the survivor in recovery begin.

As you go through the days, weeks, and months ahead, remember three key points:

1. You are not alone. Approximately 500,000 people suffer a stroke each year, and more than three million people who have had a stroke are alive today. Therefore thousands of people around the country are now caring for stroke survivors living with varying degrees of disability. In this book you'll learn how these caregivers solved many of the problems that can arise during rehabilitation and recovery.

2. You don't have to do everything yourself. During the stroke survivor's hospital stay, you probably met some of the professional staff—doctors, nurses, and therapists—who assisted in the person's medical management and early rehabilita-

tion. These professionals, and others like them, are often available to help over the long term. Even if you didn't meet these individuals, it's not too late to enlist professional help. You'll learn how in chapter 1.

In addition, other family members and friends may be happy to help you. Chapter 8 describes ways of enlisting their help so that you can take a break from caregiving.

3. You are likely to have mixed feelings about your role as caregiver. Although you are undoubtedly motivated to help, at times you will feel frustrated, angry, resentful, and depressed. These are perfectly normal feelings that usually signal the need for a break. If you accept that these "negative" feelings go hand in hand with caregiving, you won't feel guilty for experiencing them, and they won't destroy the warm, caring, and giving feelings you also have.

WHAT IS A STROKE?

A stroke is an injury to the brain that results from a sudden decrease in the flow of blood to an area of the brain, either because of a blockage from a blood clot or narrowed artery in the head or neck, or from the bursting of a section of an artery in the brain. The brain cells in the affected area become injured or die. Consequently functions normally controlled by the damaged area become impaired, either temporarily or permanently (see chapter 9 for more details).

Every person has a unique reaction to a stroke. The

effects of the stroke depend on a host of factors, from the health and personality of the survivor, to the location and severity of stroke damage in the brain, to the living arrangements and amount of support the survivor receives.

Stroke affects the survivor both physically and emotionally. After a stroke, performing even routine tasks —washing, bathing, dressing, eating, ambulating—can turn into difficult, frustrating chores that take enormous amounts of time, energy, and concentration.

The ability to communicate may be severely impaired; for example, the stroke survivor may not understand what you are saying and may not be able to speak clearly and sensibly.

Problems in thinking may also arise. These difficulties can hamper decision making, problem solving, and the ability to plan and carry out daily activities. Side effects from necessary medications such as pills to reduce high blood pressure may make these problems even more severe.

Stroke can also affect mood. The stroke survivor may experience mood swings, laugh or cry uncontrollably, feel helpless or depressed. Some stroke survivors allow others to take over the activities necessary for daily living; others strive to return to their former level of functioning and may become angry and frustrated when the body doesn't "cooperate" quickly enough.

Regardless of the extent of stroke impairment, it's crucial that the stroke survivor receive as much help and rehabilitation as possible, especially during the six months following stroke, when the body is very receptive to the kinds of training that rehabilitation can provide. You will play a vital role in the recovery process through your support, effort, and understanding.

HOW THIS BOOK CAN HELP

This book can help in three important ways. First it gives you specific techniques for helping the stroke survivor relearn lost skills and return to as normal a life as possible. You'll learn how to help with emotional, physical, behavioral, and medical problems; how to improve communication skills; and how to work effectively with rehabilitation experts and health care workers. Each chapter contains checklists and examples based on the real-life experiences of stroke survivors and their caregivers.

This book also gives you information about stroke and how damage to different parts of the brain can affect a person's personality and physical abilities. You'll gain a better understanding of the types of problems that occur, and why. You'll learn how medications can help, what to do when side effects occur, and when to call a physician. You'll also discover some of the good news about stroke treatment and rehabilitation today, namely that many people who have strokes recover and are once again able to lead rewarding, productive lives.

Finally, this book lets you know that you are not alone in your feelings, frustrations, and hopes for the future. No matter how much you want to help the person who has had the stroke, there will be times when you lose patience. This is to be expected, and should not cause feelings of guilt or inadequacy on your part.

By the same token, you have much reason for optimism. A majority of people who have experienced a stroke survive and return to independent living.

Chapter 1 covers your role in stroke recovery. You'll learn about the professional members of the stroke-recovery team, and where you fit into this group effort. In the weeks and possibly months following a stroke, professionals such as speech, physical, recreational, and occupational therapists may be available to assist the person who has had a stroke regain lost skills. You can complement the efforts of these experts by doing "home work" with the stroke survivor. In this chapter you'll also learn how to create a caregiving and recovery plan that reflects the survivor's progress in both the short and the long term.

Chapter 2 deals with emotional and behavior problems resulting from stroke, including mood swings, short attention span, anxiety, poor social judgment, and lack of "common sense" on the part of the person who has had the stroke. You'll learn ways of coping with these stressful problems to avoid losing your temper or further frustrating the stroke survivor. You'll also learn about the grieving process and how it relates to stroke recovery.

Chapter 3 covers strategies for dealing with speech and language problems, including aphasia (the inability to remember or express the names of people and common everyday objects), dysarthria (speech that is hard to understand because of weakness in the muscles that help a person speak), and apraxia (speech that is difficult to understand because of problems in the nerves that help a person put words and sentences together in the proper order).

Chapter 4 presents techniques for helping with physical problems so that the person who has experienced the stroke is as safe and comfortable as possible at home and in other environments in the community. Ways to assist the survivor in dressing, bathing, moving into and out of a wheelchair, and performing other daily activities are covered. The use of physical aids that assist in maintaining balance, ambulation, and coordination, such as a cane or walker, are also discussed.

Chapter 5 covers the medical management of stroke and its complications, including the use of medications that reduce high blood pressure or fluid retention, prevent seizures, or improve mood and behavior. Your role in helping to ensure that the stroke survivor takes the appropriate medicines will be discussed, as well as potential side effects of these medications. This chapter also includes a section on selecting a physician and other health professionals who are experienced in caring for people who have had a stroke.

Chapter 6 covers the importance of good nutrition in helping to reduce the severity of certain stroke symptoms and promote recovery. Meal planning and preparation tips for modified diets (low-fat, sodium-restricted, or calorie-restricted) are offered, as well as information on helping with chewing and swallowing problems.

Chapter 7 focuses on the role of exercise and activity in improving strength, endurance, flexibility, and coordination. You'll learn how exercise can help the stroke survivor regain skills for daily living—preparing meals, traveling, returning to work, taking up hobbies. The importance of mobility for socializing, meeting with other survivors, visiting with friends and family members, and returning to work is also discussed.

Chapter 8 offers suggestions for relieving the physical and emotional stresses of caregiving. You'll learn why taking a break is important for you and the person for whom you are caring, and specific strategies that will help prevent burnout.

Chapter 9 reviews stroke-prevention strategies and stroke warning signs. Because more than 25 percent of stroke survivors experience a second stroke, it's important to follow these strategies (many of which are part of the stroke-recovery program) and to recognize signs of a recurrent stroke. The information in this chapter may also help you and other family members avoid a stroke.

Chapter 10 includes names, addresses, and phone numbers of organizations to contact for more help and information. It also contains sections on how to obtain adaptive aids and devices for use in the home, in recreational settings, and to assist with communication problems.

Remember, stroke caregivers around the country and around the world are facing many of the same difficulties as you. By following the strategies discussed in this book and communicating with knowledgeable health professionals, you can succeed in providing vital help and support to the stroke survivor and assist in the return to a fulfilling life.

ONE

Stroke Recovery: Your Role

Ben had been in the hospital nearly a week when our doctor told me he would pull through. At first I was just so relieved. But then I felt a whole mixture of feelings. Would Ben ever be his old self again? The doctor said that while chances were good that he'd recover, there were no guarantees.

I was also terribly frightened that even if Ben did recover, it might happen again. Or what if I had a stroke? The thought was terrifying.

As for taking care of Ben, well, I admit I felt kind of trapped by all that responsibility. It didn't seem fair. I had finally retired and now I had a whole new job—caregiving—one I wasn't looking forward to at all. But when I thought that way, I started feeling guilty. I ended up resolving to take one day at a time.

—Joan

Being a caregiver for a person who has had a stroke can be a tremendously difficult job. Depending on the severity of the stroke and the length of the recovery period, the caregiving role can sap your energy, consume your time, and fill you with anxiety. No matter how much you do to help the stroke survivor, you may wonder whether it's enough. When progress is slow, you may blame yourself. And of course your own life— job, family, friends, interests—may fade as you focus large amounts of time and attention on the survivor's needs.

In this chapter we'll cover the factors that go into the decision to become a caregiver and your responsibilities during recovery. We'll also introduce you to the key recovery-team members who will serve as resources during this difficult time.

DECIDING TO BECOME A CAREGIVER

In some cases the caregiving role may be foisted upon you by circumstances, as when the person who has had a stroke is a loved one with whom you are living. Or, as the son, daughter, or other concerned relative of the stroke survivor, you may need to sit down with members of your own family and figure out how you can fit caregiving into the rest of your responsibilities. In some cases this may mean sharing the caregiving role with other relatives or friends, or seeking professional assistance. The organizations listed under "General Resources" in the Resource Guide can help you with information on health care, insurance, stroke clubs, and free or low-cost services that can make caregiving easier.

Some people are reluctant to become caregivers because, like Joan, they worry whether they are capable of doing the job. "I never really had to take care of Ben before. I always felt like he was taking care of *me,*" Joan said. But it really doesn't matter whether you have previously nursed a sick person or not. You'll learn as you go, and have the comfort of knowing that you are doing the best job you can possibly do. Nobody could ask more of any caregiver.

Your Responsibilities as Caregiver

Although you will almost certainly feel overwhelmed at times, your role in stroke recovery can also be a challenging and multifaceted one. At the beginning of the recovery period your main responsibilities will be to learn how to work with professional helpers, such as speech, physical, recreational, and occupational therapists, and to help develop a caregiving plan that can be adapted as the survivor progresses. Over the long term your primary role will be to assist the survivor in becoming as independent as possible.

When the person who has experienced the stroke returns home, you may act as his or her hands, arms, legs, or voice until mobility and speech can be regained or improved. If the survivor is receiving therapy from professionals on an outpatient basis, your "home work" will include helping with the exercises necessary to regain lost skills. If the survivor is no longer receiving regular therapy, you may still have access to professionals who can act as resources and help you feel part of a team effort.

In this chapter we'll review some of the problem areas most frequently mentioned by families and other caregivers. You'll meet the other members of the recovery team and learn how to work effectively with them during this difficult period. You'll also learn how to hire and supervise a home health care worker, who may assist you during the first few weeks after the survivor returns home.

In addition you'll learn how to adapt or develop a recovery plan that reflects the needs and progress of the person you're caring for, and your needs as well.

AFTER THE HOSPITAL: WHAT TO EXPECT

The sum total of each person's stroke-related problems can profoundly alter the pattern of day-to-day life in a family. Changes in the survivor's personality, changes in relationships, and mental and physical fatigue are the most commonly mentioned areas of concern for the caregiver, whether spouse, child, sibling, friend, or other relative. Following is an overview of what to expect in the days, weeks, and months after the survivor returns home from the hospital. These concerns, and strategies for coping with them, will be addressed in detail in the following chapters of this book.

Changes in Personality

Stroke can change the long-established behavior patterns that we associate with an individual's personality. Families often find these changes even more troubling than the physical ones. Some of the more common personality changes after a stroke can be low motivation or demanding, unreasonable behavior. Another related stroke symptom that can be of concern to the caregiver and survivor alike is emotional lability, which is the sudden, spontaneous display of an emotion such as laughing or crying. An episode can last up to several minutes and stops on its own. The frequency of emotional lability is greatest in the first few months after a stroke, and slowly abates over time.

Often a stroke survivor has difficulty processing information, which can cause him or her to misunderstand aspects of a situation and act inappropriately. Poor understanding and impulsiveness—the urge to act in a rash manner—can contribute to self-centered, demanding behavior. Also, a stroke may damage areas of the brain that have helped the person exert self-control over behavior in the past.

Caregivers can help by following the strategies set forth in the chapters to come and by setting clear limits as to what is and is not acceptable behavior. This is the only way that the survivor can begin to process information and to modify troublesome behaviors accordingly. As adults we are tuned in to subtle messages from others. The survivor may have lost some of this fine-tuning and needs the help of family and friends to know what is acceptable.

Changes in Relationships

In the weeks and months following a stroke, relationships may undergo many changes and therefore can be a source of tremendous stress. Adult children may find themselves functioning in a parental role to their own parent, or a spouse may find himself or herself functioning as a parent. The survivor may feel the helplessness and dependency often associated with childhood. He or she may feel unattractive and fear the rejection of loved ones. Sexual relationships may change. All these changes are difficult and often produce feelings of loss and grief. This is understandable, and a natural part of the process of recovering from a stroke.

Physical and Emotional Fatigue

Meeting the needs of a severely impaired stroke survivor requires an extended commitment of physical and emotional effort. Suddenly there are new demands on your time and energy in addition to the old ones. It can become very difficult to juggle all these responsibilities, and you may begin to feel pulled in too many directions at once.

We often need to remind ourselves that we are all human and that we all have limitations. We can try to do our best, given the many conflicting demands we face. By taking an occasional break from caregiving you will give yourself an opportunity to take stock, relax, and refuel. This is vital for you and for the person for whom you are caring. No caregiver can function effectively and give to others if he or she is exhausted or burdened by a sense of unreasonable guilt.

MEET THE KEY RECOVERY-TEAM MEMBERS

Fortunately in many cases you will be able to enlist the help of professionals to assist you and the survivor on the road to recovery. While the survivor was in the hospital, he or she was probably under the care of a neurologist or physiatrist and had help from other health professionals, including nurses; physical, recreational, speech, and occupational therapists; dieticians; and social workers. Some of these same professionals may be available to help you now, during the weeks and months following the immediate, or "acute," phase of rehabilitation.

"I always knew I could count on Kathleen, my husband's speech pathologist, to help us get through those long months of therapy," Lois said. "I called her whenever I had a question about the speech exercises Carl and I did at home. She always took the time to explain things to me."

Even if you no longer have access to the specific recovery-team members from the hospital, others like them may be available through resources in your community (see chapter 10). These individuals can help when problems arise over the long term.

Not every stroke-recovery team has all the members described here. The type and number of people on the team depends on several factors, including the severity of the stroke, the extent of the disabilities, and the professional personnel and facilities available in your area. Nevertheless, becoming familiar with the range of professionals who work with stroke survivors will give you a sense of the "whole picture"—and will reinforce the knowledge that you are not alone.

Neurologist

This physician, a specialist in the brain and nervous system, often heads the stroke-recovery team. Neurologists review the results of a range of physiological and cognitive tests used to determine the physical, mental, and emotional condition of the person who has had a stroke. They meet with other members of the hospital stroke-recovery team and monitor the patient's progress. Although the role of the hospital neurologist may end once the stroke survivor goes home, you may work with a neurologist in the community during the recovery process. Chapter 5 provides information on selecting the right physician(s) to monitor recovery.

Physiatrist

This physician, a specialist in physical medicine and rehabilitation, often coordinates the efforts of the health care professionals on the hospital recovery team during rehabilitation. The physiatrist is responsible for selecting appropriate therapies—physical, occupational, recreational, speech and language—for the stroke survivor. He or she also creates a preliminary list of recovery goals and a tentative time frame for recovery of some aspects of function. In many cases the physiatrist will work with the survivor's family physician in developing these goals.

Although the physiatrist's primary job ends once the stroke survivor leaves the hospital, he or she has intimate knowledge of the case and may be contacted during recovery to answer questions and give referrals.

Acute-care Nurses

Hospital acute-care nurses are among the first professionals who start stroke survivors on the road to recovery. Even before the survivor regains consciousness, the nursing staff turns him or her over in bed, takes the necessary action to prevent foot drop (a foot that dangles when the leg is lifted, because of weakness or paralysis of the ankle and foot muscles), and flexes the muscles and joints. Once the survivor is alert and starts regaining control over physical functioning, staff nurses —under the direction of the rehabilitation nurse—assist in the exercises that will help the survivor walk and move about again.

Rehabilitation Nurses

Rehabilitation nurses play an important role in the stroke survivor's recovery. They help coordinate the survivor's hospital care, administer medications, assist in urinary and bowel needs, care for the skin, and supervise the nursing staff and physical therapists to ensure that the rehabilitation plan is being followed. The rehabilitation nurse can teach you and other family members much of what you need to know to care for the stroke survivor at home.

"Before Paul left the hospital, his rehabilitation nurse taught both of us all the range-of-motion exercises, how to get him into and out of bed and into a wheelchair, how to get him to the bathroom, how to groom him—she was wonderful! She made sure we understood everything the occupational therapist and physical therapist showed us," Karen said. "She even gave us some videos and pamphlets on home care. I knew I could call her if I needed anything once Paul got home. And I did!"

Physical Therapist

Physical therapists assess the stroke survivor's movements and create a rehabilitation plan that includes specific exercises and, if needed, aids such as crutches or braces. The goal of physical therapy is to help the stroke survivor regain as much mobility, coordination, and balance as possible.

Occupational Therapist

Occupational therapists help stroke survivors regain their ability to perform everyday tasks, such as bathing, eating, dressing, cooking, and, if appropriate, driving skills and skills needed to return to work. They also help survivors adjust to problems associated with swallowing, vision, loss of sensation in the arms or legs, and perception.

The occupational therapist develops a home treatment program of exercises tailored specifically for the survivor. He or she may also do a home evaluation prior to the survivor's discharge from the hospital, and recommend the use of specific adaptive equipment, such as grab bars and wheelchair ramps.

Speech Therapist/Pathologist

Speech therapists, also known as speech pathologists, work to strengthen whatever communication skills remain after a stroke or help create a new way for the survivor to communicate (see chapter 3 for details). They will also develop a program of speech and language exercises for home use, even if the survivor continues to meet with the therapist after returning home.

"When Martin came home from the hospital, his speech was so garbled I could barely understand a word," said Peggy. "It was frustrating and also frightening. What if he was in pain or needed something and I couldn't understand him? I met with his speech pathologist who told me the daily exercises would help. They did! Within a few weeks Martin was speaking slowly, only a few words at a time, but at least I could figure out what he wanted. It was still painful, though. You never realize what you take for granted until it's taken away."

Recreational Therapist

The recreational therapist prepares a program of recreational and leisure time activities to be used by the survivor as a therapeutic part of the rehabilitation process. Recreational therapy usually includes a variety of physical and mental activities, including exercise, games, and hobbies.

Vocational Rehabilitation Specialist

A vocational rehabilitation specialist creates a program of therapeutic activities to help stroke survivors prepare for work in a specific field. The survivor may work with this professional before returning to a former job or to gain skills needed to enter a different area of employment.

Orthotist

An orthotist is a professional brace maker—the person responsible for ensuring that the survivor's braces fit properly.

Social Worker

Hospital social workers have many valuable resources at their fingertips. They may provide counseling for survivors and caregivers, information about financial assistance, and referrals to community service organizations.

"Everything was done for us. It was such a relief," said Steven. "The social workers arranged for my dad's outpatient physical and occupational therapy and found us a speech pathologist nearby. They also helped my mom understand the insurance paperwork. I know that when I go back home, my mom can call the social workers at any time and they'll be there for her. Since I have to work and can't always stay on top of everything, it's good to know that some help is available."

Psychologist

Psychologists evaluate the stroke survivor's ability to relearn lost skills and adapt to temporary and permanent disabilities. They also help the survivor cope with depression or anxiety caused by the stroke (see chapter 2 for details). Questions and problems about sexuality can also be discussed with the psychologist.

Discharge Planner

The discharge planner is the health care specialist responsible for coordinating the survivor's return to the community. He or she may arrange a home visit by a social worker or occupational therapist to determine whether adaptive equipment (e.g., guard rails, ramps) will be needed by the survivor. The discharge planner may also contact organizations in the community that can facilitate the survivor's return to an active social life (see chapter 7).

Family Physician

Your family physician should be kept informed about the survivor's progress in the hospital and upon returning home. Since the family physician is likely to coordinate the survivor's care over the long term, he or she should have access to all pertinent medical records and a list of all recovery-team members. Chapter 5 contains advice on selecting an appropriate family physician if you don't already have one or would like to change your current physician.

Guidelines for Working with the Recovery Team

As the stroke survivor's primary caregiver and an essential member of the recovery team, you are likely to be the first to recognize when something goes awry in the recovery plan. You are also in an ideal position to act as "troubleshooter"—the person who advocates for the survivor and negotiates for a better situation.

Bonnie noticed that her husband was especially irritable and distraught on the days he went to his speech therapist. When she asked Henry what was wrong, he denied having any problems. After several sessions, however, he finally told Bonnie that although the therapist had come highly recommended, he wanted to stop going. Why? The speech therapist was a man, and Henry was uncomfortable and embarrassed struggling through the exercises with him. Bonnie contacted the rehabilitation nurse, who helped her find a female speech pathologist. Now Henry is more at ease and his speech is improving.

Following are strategies for working effectively with the professional members of the recovery team to ensure that the survivor gets the best possible care:

• Schedule a time to meet with each professional helper to discuss his or her role in the recovery process and how you can help. Make these appointments even if everything is going smoothly. Then if a problem arises, you can make contact with the appropriate person quickly and don't have to spend time trying to track down the professional and introducing yourself at that time.

• If possible, bring the stroke survivor with you to the meeting. Be prepared to convey the survivor's concerns to the professional if the survivor has communication difficulties. Bring a list of questions with you that reflect your concerns as well as those of the survivor. If you meet with the professionals on your own, review the information from the meetings with the survivor when you return home.

• Consult routinely with the professional helpers about the stroke survivor's progress and whether new goals need to be set. This is especially important if rehabilitation will be a long process.

• Keep a written record of each team member's name, address, telephone number, emergency number, and office hours. Place the list by the telephone for easy access if a problem arises.

HIRING AND SUPERVISING A HOME HEALTH CARE WORKER

Immediately after returning home, and for days or even weeks afterward, the survivor may need more help than you alone can provide. You may also need time to adjust to the changes and stresses inherent in caregiving. A home health care worker can provide extra assistance during this period.

You can find a qualified home health care worker by contacting a reputable home-care nursing registry. Often the rehabilitation nurse or a hospital social worker can make recommendations or arrangements for you. You also can look under "Home Health Services" in the Yellow Pages.

If you decide to hire someone privately rather than from an agency, be aware that you are legally responsible for acting as an employer. You should check the person's licenses and references, follow state and federal payroll requirements (including payment of Social Security), and file the appropriate government forms.

Private home health care workers can be found by contacting social service agencies, churches and synagogues, or by looking in the newspaper classified-advertising section.

Be sure to check with your insurance company regarding coverage for the use of home health care workers. Many insurance plans—including Medicare—do not cover the cost of these workers.

Guidelines for Working Effectively with a Home Health Care Worker

Some home health care workers perform limited nursing or therapy tasks, while others are licensed to assist with therapeutic exercises and tasks such as feeding and bathing. Some work on a daily basis, while others live in.

Your success with a home health care worker depends on your knowing exactly what you need and expect from the person and conveying those expectations clearly from the outset. Before hiring anyone, ask yourself the following questions:

• What specific duties do I need this person to perform? *(Note:* Be aware that most home health care workers are not required to do light-housekeeping chores, and Medicare or other insurance programs may not cover such services.)
• How many hours per day and days per week do I need this individual?
• Do I need live-in help?
• Will insurance cover the cost? If not, how will I pay for this type of assistance?

You and the stroke survivor should meet with potential candidates before making a decision. This can avoid a situation such as the one Nicholas experienced:

"The agency said they had the perfect home health care worker for me. I met her and she seemed okay, but my wife, Betty, didn't meet her until the day she showed up for work. The woman was very competent, but Betty

just didn't get along with her. We had to go through the selection process all over again, but this time Betty and I interviewed the candidates together before we made a choice."

Here are some additional points to remember when bringing a home health care worker into your home:

• Make sure both you and the health care worker have a clear understanding of the chores to be done. Make a list of the agreed-upon tasks and post it in the kitchen or other area of your home.

• If the stroke survivor needs to take medications, provide the home health care worker with a written schedule to avoid confusion.

• If the health care worker is responsible for bathing the survivor, make sure he or she does so gently and thoroughly.

• If you or the stroke survivor have a conflict with a home health care worker hired from an agency, contact the personnel coordinator at the agency.

• Keep a record of the hours worked and check them against the agency's or worker's bills.

• Find out what the agency's policy is if you should find items missing from your home and you suspect the health care worker.

DEVELOPING A CAREGIVING PLAN

In the following chapters you will learn strategies and techniques for helping the stroke survivor recover and become as independent as possible. For these strategies to be most effective, they should be part of an overall caregiving plan developed by you and other members of the recovery team.

You may have spent some time creating such a plan before the stroke survivor left the hospital, in consultation with a social worker or other team members. However, even if you have already embarked on a recovery program, it will need to be reevaluated periodically to determine whether it is effective, too demanding, or not challenging enough for the survivor.

Your own needs and limitations as a caregiver will also have to be reevaluated regularly in light of your health, resources, and other responsibilities and commitments. During the weeks following a stroke you may have a substantial amount of time and energy available to help. Over the long term, however, more time and energy may need to be devoted to other obligations, such as returning to work or caring for children, and the emotional and physical stresses of caregiving may begin to take more of a toll. All these factors must be taken into consideration at various phases of recovery.

Following is an evaluation checklist to help you create a caregiving and recovery plan that is relevant to the here and now. Discuss the new plan with your physician and other health professionals to determine whether your goals are realistic and what is entailed in achieving them. This plan will need to be reevaluated from time to time.

Remember, whatever decisions you make in light of this evaluation should be based on the realities of your own situation, not on what other people think you should do or what they may have done in a similar situation. Everyone's situation is unique.

Step One: Evaluating the Caregiver's Needs and Limitations

Try to answer the following questions as honestly and completely as possible. Be aware that your situation may change over time. It's important to think ahead, as well as assess your status in the here and now.

- What other responsibilities and time commitments do you have? Include family, work, community, and recreational commitments.
- Are you physically and emotionally healthy?
- What is the extent of family financial resources, and how will they be affected by caregiving responsibilities?
- Do you need to make changes in the physical layout of your home to care for the stroke survivor? purchase and install physical aids?
- How do family members feel about caring for the stroke survivor at home?
- Will others be willing to assist in the caregiving role?
- What were the stroke survivor's relationships with family and friends before the stroke?
- How has the stroke affected those relationships?
- How do you feel about the changes in the stroke survivor?
- Are you able to spend rewarding time together?
- Have you agreed to assume caregiver responsibilities out of guilt or because you were pressured by others?
- Do you have help and support available for yourself?

In light of your responses to the above questions, try to determine the amount of time and energy you can realistically commit to the caregiving process. See chapter 10 for additional resources. Determine whether—and when—it might be appropriate to take advantage of these resources to assist in the process.

Step Two: Evaluating the Stroke Survivor's Needs and Limitations

In assessing the survivor's needs and limitations, it is important to evaluate the following areas:

Physical Abilities
Can the survivor

- Move independently whether walking or in a wheelchair?
- Control bladder and bowel functions during the day and at night? Are there special care needs such as a catheter?
- Carry out basic activities of daily living independently (dressing, personal hygiene, etc.)?
- Eat and swallow without difficulty?
- Communicate effectively (call for help if necessary)?

Cognitive Abilities
Can the survivor

- See clearly (are there perception problems)?
- Think clearly and make decisions?
- Take all necessary medications regularly?

Emotional Needs

Does the survivor

- Behave appropriately in social settings?
- Have special care needs from present or prior emotional difficulties such as depression?
- Thrive on social activity or have a strong need for privacy?

Anticipated Improvement

- What is the potential for improvement in each of the above areas? What goals can realistically be set?
- Will additional follow-up services be available (social worker, therapists) to assist in achieving these goals?

Financial Status

- What are the survivor's financial resources, including whether insurance can cover needed services?
- Is the survivor eligible for assistance through government entitlement programs, such as Medicare, Medicaid, Social Security Disability? If you are uncertain about the survivor's eligibility for government programs, contact some of the organizations, such as the American Association of Retired Persons (AARP), listed under "General Resources" in the Resource Guide.

If you have specific questions regarding Medicare, call the Social Security Administration at 1-800-234-5772.

For information about Medicaid, contact your local Human Resources Administration office. This office can also help you determine whether you are eligible for additional programs, such as food stamps.

State and local assistance programs may also be available. Check the Yellow Pages of your phone book under "Human Services" or "Human Resources" to learn about community-based, hospital-based, Veteran's Administration benefits programs and county disability programs.

Step Three: Creating a Goals-and-Progress Diary

Another helpful tool in the recovery plan is a goals-and-progress diary in which you and, if possible, the stroke survivor keep a record of progress toward specific long- and short-term goals. The diary can help give you and the survivor a sense of accomplishment over time.

Goals can be grouped into key areas such as physical goals, communication goals, family and social goals, and personal goals. Each area can include both long- and short-term areas of progress. For example:

• A long-term physical goal may be walking unaided to the store. A short-term goal may be walking across the living room to the kitchen.

• A long-term communication goal may be carrying on a conversation over the telephone. A short-term goal may be saying what you want for lunch.

• A long-term family and social goal may be going on a weekend trip to another city. A short-term goal may be going out to eat with friends.

A long-term personal goal may be to resume driving (which should only be considered after a driving evaluation has been conducted by a professional, as described in chapter 7). A short-term goal may be getting into the car and sitting behind the wheel.

All goals should be "measurable," meaning you and the survivor should be able to tell when they have been accomplished or are close to being accomplished. "Doing a better job at my leg exercises" is not measurable. "Doing five repetitions of each leg exercise" is measurable.

Keep the format simple. You may want to make a page for each day, then list each long-term goal, the short-term goals needed to accomplish it, and the steps taken that day.

As you work with the survivor, always bear in mind that each stroke is unique. Although it is helpful to read about and meet with other stroke survivors and caregivers (see chapters 7 and 8 for advice and resources), comparing the recovery of the person you're caring for with that of other stroke survivors is not recommended. Since stroke affects every person differently, it's best to focus on the progress being made in the here and now, in your own particular situation.

The following chapters will give you many specific techniques to help with the problems that arise after a stroke, including problems with emotion, behavior, communication, movement, eating, exercise, and social activities. Take your time, begin using some of these strategies, and almost before you know it, the person you are caring for will be moving along the road to recovery.

Sample Goals-and-Progress Diary

Today's date: 1/31/94
Long-term Goal: To resume driving
Short-term goals: To get to the car unaided, open the door and get into the vehicle, know all the instruments on the dashboard, start the car, shift gears, use rearview mirror to back out of driveway.
Today's accomplishments:

1. Walked to the car
2. Opened the door
3. Got into the vehicle unaided
4. Sat in the car for several minutes
5. Held on to the steering wheel
6. Tried to name all the items on the dashboard.

Comments: Slipped and fell while walking. Needed both hands to open door. Felt good to hold on to the steering wheel. Still can't remember the name of the thing that tells how many miles you've gone.

TWO

Helping with Mood and Behavior Problems

Sometimes Connie cries for no apparent reason and then suddenly stops. It drives me crazy. I don't know what to do. Most of the time I just ignore it. But what if something is really wrong?

—*Sam*

My father used to be reserved and quiet. Now he interrupts people during a conversation and bullies his way into their business. I'm embarrassed to be with him when he's like this.

—*Susan*

Harriet has lost all interest in her friends and in music, two things she enjoyed before her stroke. Now she just wants to watch television, and she doesn't call her friends back when they call her. I try to persuade her to be sociable. But she seems so depressed that I'm starting to feel depressed too.

—*Irv*

A stroke can cause many bewildering changes in the survivor's emotions and behavior. Suddenly the man or woman you married—or your mother, father, or other close relative—may seem like a different person. In a way such people are different; their brains have been injured and the behaviors and emotions they display are a reflection of that injury.

These changes can be unsettling, causing you to wonder whether your relationship with the survivor will ever be the same as it was before the stroke. In many cases caregivers and others react to this relationship "loss" with a form of grief that encompasses various stages. At the same time they must cope with the changes in the survivor and help the survivor to cope and recover. This can be a trying process, but knowing what to expect can help everyone involved move through this difficult period.

In this chapter we'll explore the grieving process that follows when survivors and caregivers begin to comprehend their personal losses. We'll also look at the ways in which the injuries to the brain incurred from a stroke affect emotions and behavior. These insights will provide a basis for understanding that many of the inappropriate things that the survivor may say or do are a result of injury—not purposeful attempts to provoke you.

THE GRIEVING PROCESS

People who experience a loss—whether from death, divorce, or an accident or illness that renders a previously healthy individual helpless or deficient in their ability to function—react in similar ways. These reactions have been described in stages, and form what is called the grieving process. The closer you have been to a person affected by stroke, the more likely you are to experience some of these feelings.

The stages of grieving are neither inevitable nor necessarily sequential. One stage doesn't abruptly stop so that the next can begin. Rather, grieving is a gradual healing process that takes time and work. You may move back and forth among the stages at your own pace. And although "coping" is the last stage, you are likely to cope with the situation to some extent throughout the process.

Stage One: Shock

"I must be dreaming. This can't really be happening to us!"

Feelings of numbness, unreality, confusion, and fear may be experienced by caregivers and survivors alike after a stroke has occurred. Many people also feel helpless. The support of family and friends is crucial at this time.

Stage Two: Denial

"The doctors don't know what they're talking about. My wife will be up and around just like new in a few weeks."

Denial is the way we avoid facing the overwhelming reality of a devastating situation. It is positive in that it sets up a goal—full recovery—but in this stage you may not acknowledge the steps necessary to reach that goal. Nevertheless focusing on recovery can help propel you and the survivor into the next stage.

Stage Three: Reaction

"My life is destroyed. Nothing will ever be the same."

When you begin to accept that the stroke and the resulting disabilities are a reality, depression often sets in. In fact some family members and survivors may feel so devastated, they believe death would have been preferable to living with the dysfunctions they now face. This is a very normal reaction; do not feel guilty about feeling this way. It is part of the grieving process.

Other common reactions, which may go hand in hand with depression, are anger and frustration.

"I used to think, 'How could my husband do this to me?' I know the stroke wasn't his fault, yet I wanted to blame someone."

Again, these feelings are normal—not a cause for guilt or self-recrimination. Only after mourning the loss of the person he or she knew can a caregiver learn who that person has become and begin to develop a comfortable relationship. It is a slow process that is difficult for the caregiver—especially a spouse—and for the survivor, who must begin to know a new self.

Stage Four: Mobilization

This is the action stage, when stroke survivors say, "I'm ready to learn how to beat this thing," and caregivers may become more motivated to help in the recovery process. In this stage it is important to acknowledge how far the caregiver and survivor have come and to start looking ahead realistically.

Stage Five: Coping

This is the final stage of the healing process, when the caregiver and survivor learn to live with the disabilities the stroke has caused.

"I take each day as it comes and live it to its fullest," says Rhonda, whose husband is in a wheelchair six months after his stroke. "We plan short trips. If George feels up to it, we go. If not, we always have an alternate plan. You can't let it get you down!"

Remember, there are no set time limits for any of these stages. You reach the coping stage when you are ready—and even then you may move back into earlier stages for brief periods. Respect your feelings and allow yourself to grieve and heal at your own pace.

WHAT TO DO ABOUT DEPRESSION

As we've seen, depression or despair is a normal part of the grieving process, for both the caregiver and the survivor. However, sometimes depression can become serious enough to impair functioning. It is important to identify the warning signs of depression (see sidebar, page 32) so that steps may be taken to alleviate it.

If the caregiver becomes seriously depressed, he or she may not be able to continue caring for the survivor during this period.

"I realized something was wrong when I visited Mom and Dad," Barbara said. "Mom looked as though she hadn't been bathed in days. And when I asked Dad what was happening, he shrugged his shoulders. 'What's the difference whether she has a bath or not? She still can't talk or eat right. This stroke has ruined us. Trying to make anything better seems hopeless.' I realized Dad was really depressed, and I called our family doctor. He ended up prescribing medication and also suggesting that we have a housekeeper come in for a few weeks to help out."

If the stroke survivor becomes seriously depressed, the caregiver should take steps to ensure that treatment is obtained.

"Roger was so vital and active before his stroke," explained his wife, Bernadette. "He supervised twenty people at work, played tennis once a week, and was head of the finance committee at church. After he came home from the rehabilitation hospital, he showed no interest in anything. Getting him to do his exercises was a real struggle. 'What's the use?' he'd say. 'I'll never be what I was before.' He wouldn't let anyone visit him, and he wouldn't go out, even though the church com-

mittee urged him to come to the meetings. Finally I called the social worker and she referred us to a psychologist. Until we dealt with the depression, it didn't look like we were going to get anywhere with Roger's therapy."

Getting Through Depression

One way to deal with depression is to seek counseling with a social worker, psychologist, or other trained health professional. Members of the stroke-recovery team (see chapter 1) may act as resources or refer you to an appropriate professional.

Other strategies can also be effective. One technique for dealing with your own depression is to change your behavior. By behaving differently you may actually improve your mood. For example, doing something active, such as taking an exercise class or going for a walk, can help break a depressive mood that leaves you sitting around doing nothing.

Caregivers and stroke survivors alike have found that some of the most effective tools for combatting depression involve goal setting and time structuring. Having a daily activity schedule can provide structure, a feeling of organization, and a sense of purpose for you and for the survivor. See chapter 1 for advice on setting up a goals-and-progress diary that can pave the way for moving out of a slump and forging ahead.

To help the survivor overcome depression, try some of the following tips:

• In consultation with your physician, help relieve the physical problems that may be contributing to

Warning Signs of Depression

According to the *American Psychiatric Association Diagnostic and Statistical Manual,* criteria for the diagnosis of depression include

- Changes in appetite and weight
- Disturbed sleep (for example, not being able to sleep through the night)
- Motor agitation or retardation (for example, constantly fidgeting or moving slowly and lethargically)
- Fatigue and loss of energy
- Depressed or irritable mood
- Loss of interest or pleasure in usual activities
- Feelings of worthlessness, self-reproach, or excessive guilt
- Suicidal thinking or attempts
- Difficulty thinking or concentrating

If at least five of these nine criteria are present, a diagnosis of major depressive illness, or clinical depression, may be made by a physician.

depression, such as pain, muscle spasms, or constipation.

- Encourage the survivor to spend some time each day doing something he or she enjoys, whether it is listening to music, doing puzzles, or simply taking in the view outside your window.
- Encourage the survivor to participate in social ac-

tivities. If mobility is a problem, invite friends over to play cards, watch a video, or have dinner with the survivor.

• Praise the survivor for accomplishments and acknowledge progress. Positive words can enhance self-confidence, self-esteem, and a good self-image.

• Include the survivor in family decision making. Even if he has trouble understanding everything you discuss, it's important for him to know he is still part of the family.

• Avoid using phrases such as "cheer up" or "it could be worse." These expressions, which discount the survivor's feelings, can make the person feel even more depressed.

• Medications to treat depression may be prescribed by a physician (see chapter 5 for details).

RESUMING SEXUAL ACTIVITY

The quality of a couple's sexual relationship following a stroke differs from couple to couple. The closeness that you shared before the stroke can often be the best indicator of how your relationship will evolve after a stroke. Remember that sexual satisfaction, both giving and receiving, can be accomplished in many ways. Whatever is comfortable and acceptable to both partners is normal.

Many husbands and wives of stroke survivors worry that sexual activity may cause another stroke or result in other damage. No studies have shown this to be true. Individuals who had a hemorrhagic stroke, however, should check with their physician before resuming sexual activities.

Some male stroke survivors experience impotence (inability to have or sustain an erection), which may be caused by the depression that often occurs after a stroke. Given time, patience, and perhaps counseling, impotence can resolve. If the wife is the stroke survivor, the husband may experience impotence because he is afraid he will hurt his wife. Often the best approach is for the couple to talk about their needs and fears with each other or a counselor who can help them deal with their concerns.

Sometimes medication can cause impotence. If the male stroke survivor has no morning erection and is taking diuretics, tranquilizers, antidepressants, sedatives, blood pressure medication, or heart medication, the drugs may be causing the decreased sex drive. Contact your physician about this situation (see chapter 5).

The presence of catheters need not stop sexual activity. Both men and women can remove, clamp, or disconnect an external collecting device or internal catheter. Your physician or occupational therapist can show you how.

Of course the presence of medical paraphernalia, combined with weakness or uncertainty on the part of the afflicted partner, can cause the caregiver to lose sexual interest. On the other hand the stroke survivor may have difficulty feeling sexual desire for the caregiver, who has essentially taken on a mothering role.

The best approach is to talk to each other about your feelings. Sometimes honest discussion can "break the ice" enough to permit desire to surface. You can also try being playful with each other, especially as you remove an item such as a catheter. Playing music, turning down the lights, and doing whatever else helps you create a romantic environment (think back to particularly pleasurable prestroke sexual encounters) can encourage sexual expression.

EFFECTS OF RIGHT-BRAIN INJURY ON MOOD AND BEHAVIOR

When the right side of the brain is injured, the left side of the body is often paralyzed to some degree. Since the right hemisphere controls emotions, nonverbal communication, and spatial orientation (sense of body position), damage to this side of the brain may cause an array of emotion and behavior problems.

People with right-side brain injury may experience emotional highs and lows (emotional lability), short attention span, poor judgment (especially regarding their own safety), confused thinking, memory loss, lack of motivation and interest, impulsiveness, and impaired abstract thinking.

They may also have trouble judging distances, size, position, rate of movement, forms, and how parts relate to a whole. These are known as spatial-perceptual deficits, and they can make it difficult for stroke survivors to maneuver in or relate to their environment.

These deficits may overlap in people with right-side brain injury, causing multiple problems. For example, when Robert decided he could go up the stairs without his cane and without asking anyone for help, he showed poor judgment and was acting impulsively. Once he reached the stairs, his inability to judge distances prevented him from placing his foot on the bottom stair. This was fortunate, for if he had begun climbing, he probably would have fallen. Impatient with himself, he began cursing, which led his wife to come running in from the other room. She successfully maneuvered him away from the stairway.

Emotional Highs and Lows

Some stroke survivors spontaneously burst into laughter or crying spells that last up to several minutes. This condition, called *emotional lability,* is a physical condition that is greatest in the first few months after a stroke and slowly abates over time. It is important to realize that there is often no relationship between the fact that the person is crying and what is happening in the environment. Nor can you assume that crying is a display of emotion reflecting the survivor's true feelings at the time.

"A few months after Mike had his stroke, we were in a restaurant and suddenly he began laughing and shouting. I was so embarrassed," said his wife, Martha. "He stopped after a minute. I knew he didn't realize what he was doing, but it's still hard to deal with." Mike repeated this behavior several times in the next few months. Martha is happy to report that it hasn't happened again in more than a year. "I don't know if he'll ever do it again. At least I know our family and friends understand if he does."

Coping Strategies

Emotional lability and outbursts can be very trying for the caregiver. Here are ways to curtail such behavior:

• Interrupt the behavior by distracting the survivor's attention. If he or she immediately stops crying when you change the subject or call his or her name, this is a sign that the emotional outburst is probably due to brain damage from the stroke rather than sadness or depression.

• Accept the behavior in a matter-of-fact way. Continue the conversation or activity and ignore the display of emotion.

• If the survivor apologizes, accept the apology and acknowledge, "This is a symptom of stroke." This will diminish any embarrassment and permit current activities to continue.

Short Attention Span

Right-brain injury often causes survivors to have short attention and retention spans. They may be cooking something on the stove and then simply walk away and start doing something else. Any distraction—background music, other people in the room—will cause them to lose concentration.

"Janet was always so capable. She never undertook any project, from helping with a church fund-raiser to planning our vacation, unless she knew she could see it through," Dan said. "Now she jumps from chore to chore, never finishing what she started. If I ask why she

stopped, she says she just doesn't feel like doing it anymore. She can't seem to plan ahead even a day in advance."

Coping Strategies

To help the survivor stay focused on the task at hand, try the following:

• Keep the environment as quiet as possible. Turn the television and radio off and unplug the telephone.

• Divide tasks into steps. For example if the survivor is relearning how to do the laundry, start with separating clothes into colors and whites, then placing them in the laundry bag, taking them to the machine, adding detergent, and so forth.

• Give positive feedback during and between steps.

• Encourage the survivor to slow down when she starts to move or react too quickly. Let her know that you can wait while she does a task step-by-step.

• Supervise any project that may be harmful if the survivor tends to walk away, such as cooking or ironing.

Poor Judgment

Right-brain injury may also cause survivors to use poor judgment and overestimate their abilities. They may try such feats as attempting to walk across a room without using their brace or to pick up a glass with a paralyzed hand. Some of the attempts can be life-threatening, as when Abigail tried to drive her husband's car. Mark was in the study reading when he heard a crash and discovered that his wife had taken the car keys, backed the car down the driveway, and run over the mailbox before coming to a stop. Luckily she was unhurt.

"I call it the 'superman complex,'" says Dorothy. "Sometimes my father insists he can dance. The truth is, he can barely walk. But when he makes this claim, I make sure I'm right there next to him in case he tries!"

Coping Strategies

Knowing that the survivor has impaired judgment can be very anxiety-provoking to the caregiver. For safety's sake:

• Don't overestimate survivors' abilities, no matter how much she tries to convince you of her capabilities.
• If the survivor insists he or she can perform complex tasks, stay with the person and monitor the activity.

Confused Thinking and Memory Loss

For some stroke survivors, planning and carrying out even the simplest activities may cause confusion.

"I walked into our bedroom and my husband was standing there with his pants on, but he was holding his underwear in his hand," said Stephanie. "He simply couldn't remember what he was supposed to do with it."

Coping Strategies

In the spirit of helping the survivor become as independent as possible, try the following techniques for simplifying tasks and activities:

• Just as for survivors with short attention spans, confusion is minimized if you write out step-by-step directions for tasks such as getting dressed, doing the laundry, or making a sandwich. For survivors who cannot follow written directions, make a picture board showing the sequence of steps they should follow.

• Establish fixed routines whenever possible. Do you have meals at set times? Are there certain days or times the grandchildren call? Do you treat yourselves to pizza every Friday night? Big or small, established events or traditions can help survivors orient themselves and feel more secure.

• Present new information slowly and one step at a time.

• Give the survivor frequent feedback about his or her progress.

• Use memory aids such as schedule cards, appointment books, and calendars. Posting notes or pictures around the house as reminders can be particularly helpful. For example when Beverly's father had trouble remembering where certain food items were in the kitchen, she cut out pictures of cereal, milk, cheese, bread, fruit, and other foods and taped them to the refrigerator and cabinets. This lessened his dependence on his daughter and increased his feeling of independence.

Lack of Interest or Motivation

Stroke survivors who lack motivation or interest in people and situations around them are often depressed. Treatment of the depression usually restores interest and enthusiasm.

Spatial-Perceptual Problems

Have you ever thought there was one more step on a staircase and been surprised when your foot "missed" it? Have you ever misjudged the edge of a table and dropped your spoon in your lap? If so, you've made spatial-perceptual errors.

Problems with performing spatial-perceptual tasks (those requiring ability to judge size, rate of movement, distance, position, and form) are common among stroke survivors with right-side brain injury. Survivors with this impairment have trouble performing tasks that require them to determine how big or small something is, how fast it is moving, what shape it is, or how far away it is from them. They may not be able to tell the difference between right and left or whether they are sitting or standing. When they read, they quickly lose their place on the page. They may button a shirt incorrectly or put a dress on inside out. When maneuvering their wheelchair through a doorway, they may run it into the doorjamb.

One specific type of perceptual problem experienced by stroke survivors is called *agnosia*—an inability to interpret what they touch, see, smell, taste, or hear. They may know they are holding a quarter in their hand but not be able to tell you its weight, shape, or size.

"My brother tried to brush his teeth with a pencil," said Herb. "We had to take all the medicines and cleaning supplies out of the cabinets when he tried to drink the detergent, thinking it was a bottle of soda."

Another type of problem is *one-sided neglect,* when the survivor loses a portion of his or her sight. It feels as though he is wearing swimming goggles with half of each lens covered. As a result a man may only shave the right half of his face or a woman may only put lipstick on the right side of her mouth. This was the case with Heidi's father. When Heidi noticed that he ate food only on one side of his plate, she suggested that he always turn his plate around when he thinks he has finished so that he can see the other side.

Stroke survivors with right-brain injury may also lose vision in the left field or unconsciously neglect the left limbs in the environment.

General Tips for Dealing with Problems Related to Right-Brain Injury

Because stroke survivors with right-brain injury often don't have the speech and communication problems that affect people with left-brain injury, their spatial-perceptual difficulties are sometimes overlooked. When these individuals begin having trouble performing simple activities, they may be labeled uncooperative, overly dependent, confused, or unmotivated. Once caregivers and family members realize spatial-perceptual difficulties are the cause, they can help stroke survivors better deal with this problem:

• Keep the environment safe. Like Herb, you may need to keep all potentially dangerous items, such as sharp objects, cleaning agents, and poisons, out of the survivor's reach.

• Monitor the survivor's activities. If left unattended, she may become confused or injure herself.

• Arrange the environment to allow for visual and sensory problems. If individuals cannot perceive things on their left side, place items they need on their right. For example, place clothes on the right side of closets and drawers.

• Encourage survivors to acknowledge the affected half of their body as a part of them. Some people give their paralyzed arm or leg a nickname, as if it were a separate entity. Individuals who feel this way must be reminded that the affected side of their body is part of them, too, and needs their care and attention.

• Give frequent reminders of the affected side by touching it, rubbing it, or asking the survivor to massage it. Wearing a visual reminder on the affected arm or leg, such as a bracelet, watch, or bright shoelaces, can remind survivors to pay attention to that part of their body.

• Encourage them to scan—turn their head from side to side—in order to see what they usually ignore on the affected side. Point out landmarks as you walk or travel in order to give them a reason to scan.

• Some people with agnosia lose their sense of direction and may get lost, even in their own homes. Never leave them alone where they may wander off. Get an identification bracelet or pendant to wear with their name, your name, address, and phone number in case they do wander off when you are not watching them.

• Minimize clutter in the stroke survivor's environment. Too much visual and auditory stimulation can add to his or her confusion and may be dangerous.

• Prevent injuries caused by the individual's inability to determine depth and distance by clearly marking pointed edges on furniture, doorways, and other items.

EFFECTS OF LEFT-BRAIN INJURY ON MOOD AND BEHAVIOR

When the left side of the brain is injured, the right side of the body is often paralyzed to some degree. This side of the brain controls language and verbal communication in most people, and consequences of damage in that area will be covered in detail in the next chapter. Damage to the left side of the brain can also cause personality changes; survivors with left-brain damage tend to behave in a cautious, compulsive, or disorganized way and are easily frustrated. These behaviors and emotional responses may be related to speech and language problems, in that the survivor is slow to respond to questions or to take action.

Cautious, Compulsive Behavior

When left-brain damage causes slowness or caution, you may feel impatient with the survivor. Although this is a normal feeling, it's important to remember that he is not being purposefully obstinate. Rather he is probably attempting to orient himself and feel more secure.

"My father used to be full of get-up-and-go. Some nights after work he would take courses at the local community college. On weekends he would be out gardening or taking in a baseball game," said Shawn. "Now he sits around all the time, like he's afraid to go out. All he does is watch the same television programs day after day."

Coping Strategies

To help promote the survivor's sense of confidence and security, try the following:

• Give plenty of encouragement and positive feedback for accomplishments. Use words like "that's right," "good," and "you're doing fine."
• If the person has difficulty understanding speech, then smile, nod reassuringly, and pat the individual on the back or arm to show support.

Easily Frustrated

When survivors with left-brain damage are thwarted in their efforts to communicate or perform simple tasks, they may become frustrated and give up.

Coping Strategies

To motivate the survivor to continue with the task at hand:

• Show that you are paying attention and willing to help. This will often motivate the survivor to continue.

• Give praise, verbal and nonverbal, for each accomplishment.

Apraxia

Apraxia is the inability voluntarily to perform certain skilled movements despite adequate muscle strength. In other words the person is able to perform the movement when not thinking about it but cannot do so if asked.

There are several different manifestations of apraxia, named for the functions that are affected by the impairment. For example, with motor apraxia, the person may be physically able to stand up but unable to do so if asked.

Another kind of apraxia is dressing apraxia. The survivor may be unable to put on a sweater if asked, but may later slip it on without thinking or may put on clothes inappropriately, such as upside down or inside out.

Apraxia can lead to misunderstandings between the stroke survivor and caregivers. What appears to be stubbornness or manipulative behavior may be a symptom of apraxia instead.

Coping Strategies

To help the survivor with apraxia:

• Talk the person through the activity, guiding the hand and demonstrating the desired movement.

• Phrase instructions so that they refer to a goal

rather than to the steps to achieve the goal. For example if you tell a survivor to "stand up," he or she may not be able to do so. But if you ask her to "please come into the living room," she can respond. "Put your coat on" may be more effective than "put your arm in the sleeve."

• Remember that apraxia is the result of damage to the brain, in particular the parts that allow people to translate ideas into action. It is not purposefully obstinate behavior.

General Tips for Dealing with Problems Related to Left-Brain Injury

Mood and behavior changes associated with left-brain injury can be frustrating to the survivor and caregiver alike. To assist the survivor in his or her attempts to perform as normally as possible:

• Be patient. Give the survivor time to think about each step involved in a task or problem solving. Don't rush him.

• Give immediate and frequent feedback—verbally, with gestures, or both. Focus on the positive. Avoid statements such as "Why did you do that?" or "When are you going to get it right?"

• Keep questions and comments simple. Questions should be stated so that the survivor can give a yes-or-no answer.

• Speak in a normal voice unless you know the individual has a hearing problem.

In the next chapter we'll present many specific strategies that have been shown to be effective in helping the survivor with communication problems resulting from left- and right-brain injury. Using these techniques can help lessen the anxiety and frustration you may feel when attempting to understand and meet the needs of the survivor.

THREE

Helping with Communication Problems

When Emma first came home, it was like a night-mare. She couldn't talk, or write. I didn't know what to think. Even though they told me her mental abilities were intact, it was hard to believe she could still think and feel. I was frustrated even trying to figure out when she was hungry or thirsty, or had to go to the bathroom.

Then, after a few days, I got the idea that maybe she could peck at my computer with the fingers of her good hand. Was I relieved when it worked! It was as though she could suddenly talk again. And when she did really start talking a few weeks later, she told me how much my patience had meant to her.

Now Emma is her old self again. But I'll never forget the fear and frustration of that first week.

—Ken

How do you feel when a word or phrase is "right on the tip of your tongue" but won't come to you? Or when your speech is slurred after the dentist gives you a shot of novocaine? Are you frustrated? Embarrassed? Angry?

This is what life can feel like for the stroke survivor whose communication skills are impaired. For most of us these are temporary conditions. If we can't find the right word, we use another; we know the dentist's novocaine will wear off soon. But for stroke survivors, however, communication problems may take months or years to resolve.

In this chapter we'll look at some of the common communication problems that may follow a stroke, including *aphasia*—loss of the power to speak, write, gesture, or comprehend spoken, written, or gestured language; *dysarthria*—slurred, slow, imprecise speech; *apraxia*—the inability voluntarily to produce specific words or sounds; and *pragmatic deficit*—excessive or inappropriate speech. Coping strategies and activities you can use to better understand the survivor and facilitate communication with others are included.

UNDERSTANDING COMMUNICATION

Communication is the sharing of experiences, thoughts, ideas, and feelings through verbal and nonverbal means. Communication encompasses the use of speech and language—including grammar and vocabulary—as well as sounds and gestures.

Pragmatics is the technical term used to describe nonverbal communication skills, including the understanding and use of nonverbal cues, such as tone of voice and facial expression, and proper interpretation of social situations. Pragmatics allow a person to know what to say to whom, and when and how it is appropriate to say it. One problem that can result from stroke is called pragmatic deficit, meaning that the survivor may misread nonverbal cues and talk in socially inappropriate ways, such as trying to take over a conversation or going off on tangents (see page 62).

Communication breakdowns may occur at any stage of receiving or sending a message in one or all of the above categories. The types of communication problems that result from stroke depend on the part of the brain affected and the severity of the damage.

EFFECTS OF LEFT-BRAIN INJURY ON COMMUNICATION

Damage to the left side of brain may result in communication disorders affecting listening, speaking, reading, and writing.

Aphasia

Imagine if every time someone talked to you, all you heard were garbled noises. Or if you wanted to say the word *car* but something else, such as the word *man* or a string of nonsense syllables, came out instead.

Left-brain injury may cause an inability to express *(expressive aphasia)* or understand *(receptive aphasia)* spoken or written words. Survivors have described a feeling similar to running through a maze in their mind, searching for an elusive word or misplaced thought.

Phil explains how his wife sometimes launches into a long series of thoughts before she can find the word she wants:

"Phil, where is the cooking thing?"

"What 'thing,' Clare?"

"You know, the thing we put food into."

"You mean the frying pan?"

"No, it's bigger than that."

"The skillet?"

"No, this is taller."

"Is it round?"

"What?"

"Like this?" (Phil makes a circle with his arms.)

"Yes, yes it is."

"The spaghetti pot?"

"Yes, that's it!"

Aphasia may cause survivors to speak in gibberish, although they believe they are making sense. Or they may use automatic speech—common social words and phrases such as "hello," "nice day," or "good-bye"—to reply to any comments directed to them, simply because these are the only words they can access and verbalize.

"How are you today, Mary?"

"Fine."

"Did you have your lunch yet?"

"Fine."

"Did Peggy come in to see you today?"

"Fine."

Profane language may be used in the same way. Be aware that the use of such words has no meaning to people with aphasia; they could just as easily be saying *cake* or *house*.

Individuals with aphasia may be able to understand words but not be able to write, read, or say them. They may not be able to interpret pictures or symbols. These limitations may range in severity. Some survivors only occasionally misunderstand a word, while others are unable to understand any speech at all.

It is not possible to say with certainty how quickly or how much the person with aphasia will improve. The reason is that aphasia is the result of problems with memory, not with language itself. In other words the survivor is not relearning language; he or she is waiting for memory to return, and many of the exercises used by speech therapists and pathologists are designed to help stimulate memory.

Because most people with aphasia are intellectually unimpaired, the disorder can be extremely frustrating for all concerned. Survivors with aphasia may withdraw from conversations to avoid frustration or to avoid "bothering" other people. But keeping the person engaged in family conversations and interactions is a vital part of recovery. The survivor will feel motivated to continue to improve while experiencing the much-needed comfort of being part of the family.

Coping Strategies

A speech pathologist can prepare appropriate exercises for therapy sessions and work at home. In addition there are simple techniques you can use at home to help stimulate the survivor's ability to use speech and language:

• Encourage the survivor to point to objects or make gestures to show you what he or she wants.

• Make a word or picture board, as Charles did when he became frustrated with his wife, Doris. At first Charles would ask, "What do you want for dinner?" and name several items. Doris would struggle to respond and end up gesturing wildly. So the speech therapist suggested that Charles collect food labels and cut out pictures of food from magazines, then mount these on a board. Now Doris simply points to the food she prefers. Charles reinforces each selection by naming the items out loud each time she makes a choice.

• Speak clearly and concisely, communicating one idea at a time. Long, complex sentences are difficult for people with aphasia to understand. "Bobby and I went to the store yesterday and bought some new plants for the front yard and patio" is far too complicated. Three shorter sentences with pauses in between are more likely to be understood. "Bobby and I went shopping." "We bought some plants." "We put them in the yard."

• Phrase questions so that they require only a yes-or-no answer. "Do you want to eat now?" "Would you like a glass of iced tea?"

• Use gestures to help explain what you are saying. For example, as you say "Do you want to wear the red blouse?" point to the blouse and mimic putting it on.

• Attempt to understand invented words and phrases. Barbara utters words that approximate the ones she means. For example she says "pabble I" for apple pie and "sandbury moose" for cranberry juice. Since Barbara has no control over these speech patterns, she and her family simply accept what her daughter has dubbed "creative phrases."

• See whether the survivor responds to music. For example, Mort was pleasantly surprised when his mother, who had spoken only a few words in the two months following her stroke, starting singing "Spanish Eyes" one day while the song played on the radio. "She got all the words right!" he said enthusiastically. Yet after the song was over, so was Hazel's debut. She still could not say what she wanted. The speech pathologist explained that while speech is controlled by the left side of the brain, music is interpreted on the right side, which was unaffected. Music therapy combined with mime was added to Hazel's speech program.

Assessing Progress

If you have questions about the survivor's speech and language abilities, talk with your speech and language therapist. Some of the tests that are generally administered in the hospital to determine how well the survivor can understand, speak, write, and read may be given again to assess improvement. One of these tests is called the Functional Communication Profile, which is an informal interview used to measure a person's ability to communicate in everyday situations. Many communication parameters are assessed, including whether the person can indicate yes or no and whether he can say his own name or recognize the names of friends and family members.

Another test is the Token Test, which measures depth of understanding of spoken language. The test consists of a series of verbal directions to perform tasks with various colored shapes. For example the survivor may be asked to "put the blue square on the red circle," or "touch the green square." The test is often used to track communication progress over time.

Dysarthria

Left-brain injury may cause damage to the area that controls the muscles used in speech. The result is dysarthria—weakness, slowness, or lack of coordination of the muscles involved in producing speech (in the chest, lips, tongue, vocal folds, and jaw). People with dysarthria know what they want to say but lack the fine-muscle control necessary to produce clear speech. Like other deficits, dysarthria may range in severity, causing occasional slurring of sounds, the production of "mushy"-sounding words, slow and monotonous speech, or, at the extreme, speech may become completely unintelligible.

Coping Strategies

To help the survivor with dysarthria make himself or herself understood:

• Encourage the person to slow down when speaking. One way to accomplish this is to have the survivor tap his or her fingers on the table while pronouncing each syllable.

• Help the survivor practice breath control (usually taught by a speech therapist). Encouraging deep, regular breathing helps the survivor regulate the physical aspects of speaking, such as breathing in before saying words rather than afterward. It also reduces the tendency to speak too loudly.

Verbal Apraxia

Verbal apraxia occurs when the muscles that produce speech are intact but the brain's ability to send messages telling the muscles to move a certain way in order to voluntarily produce specific sounds is impaired. The commands get mixed up and out of order. Consider Larry's dilemma: Most of the time, he says his words slowly but correctly. However, occasionally a word doesn't come out the way he intended. For example, he knows he wants to say "look," but his tongue won't rise up to the roof of his mouth to form the el; instead a pee sound comes out, making the word sound like "pook." He may continue to try, only to have an ess sound come out. After several attempts he can usually say the word he has in mind.

Certain sounds are more difficult than others for people with apraxia, and the degree of difficulty appears to follow a developmental pattern—that is, the order in which children learn to speak. Words such as *ma* and *pa* are among the first that children learn, and these are the easiest words for survivors with apraxia to say. Blends—two syllables together, such as *br* or *pl*—which require more verbal skills, are the most difficult to relearn. Speech-therapy exercises follow the same pattern, moving from the simpler sounds to the more complicated ones. Computer programs that feature word drills and provide the user with feedback (i.e., whether their speech is correct or incorrect) can be used in addition to regular sessions with a speech therapist. See the Resource Guide for companies that supply these programs.

Coping Strategies

Speech-improvement exercises are the cornerstone of progress with verbal apraxia:

• Help the survivor practice words and letter combinations until they are pronounced correctly and as intended.

• If the person can write better than he or she can speak, encourage this means of communication while continuing to do speech-improvement exercises.

• If you can afford to purchase a home computer or rent one several times a week, the survivor can use speech-therapy software to practice independently and receive feedback.

Reading Problems

Some survivors may lose much or all of their ability to read and comprehend written words. Others may understand single sentences but not entire paragraphs. Some lose the ability to understand "little" words (such as *is, not, he, she, it)*; still others omit or add so many words that they lose the meaning of what they are reading entirely.

Coping Strategies

Loss of the ability to read can be extremely frustrating to survivors, especially for those who enjoyed reading prior to the stroke. To motivate the survivor to continue attempting to read despite comprehension problems:

• Suggest stimulating reading material, such as popular novels or even young adult fiction. Mysteries and action-adventure stories with strong story lines can keep the survivor interested and absorbed to the point where the inability to understand every single word becomes less of a deterrent.

• Allow for reduced attention span by arranging frequent breaks. Some survivors may find they can read only a paragraph or two at a time before taking a rest.

• Encourage overall comprehension rather than focusing on every single word. Those who miss the "little" words may still be able to understand enough of the bigger words to make sense of an article or story.

• Use books on tape or video as less stressful alternatives, while continuing to encourage reading.

Writing Problems

When Claudia could not understand what her aunt was trying to tell her, she gave her a pencil and paper and asked her aunt to write the word. After several minutes her aunt managed to scrawl the letters bossroo.

"Bossroo?" Claudia exclaimed. "But that's the same thing you've been saying. I still don't know what that means."

A survivor's ability to write will be affected by the type of brain damage he or she has sustained. Survivors with aphasia, such as Claudia's aunt, will be unable to write words they cannot say. The reason is that the problem is their inability to think of the word they want; if they think "bossroo," that's what they will write. A survivor may also lose the knowledge of how to make the letters of the alphabet, or his or her ability to spell.

On the other hand if a survivor has dysarthria or verbal apraxia, his ability to write may be unimpaired.

When stroke affects the right side of the brain and results in spatial-perceptual problems, some individuals may have trouble writing because they cannot determine direction and space. They may write words and sentences on top of one another or write all over the page without regard to lines or margins.

Coping Strategies

Writing problems can result from memory problems or physical problems. In either case it helps to:

• Have the survivor spend some time writing every day. Encourage the person to take his or her time and to take frequent rests.

• Suggest that she write about something of interest, such as describing the family pet or a favorite hobby she hopes to resume. The survivor can also complete the daily-progress diary outlined in chapter 1.

• Play word games that involve the survivor's saying the names of specific items you point to and then writing down the names.

Computation

People with aphasia often have trouble performing activities that require computation skills (work with numbers). They may write a check correctly but not know how to subtract the amount to figure the new balance. Or they may not be able to calculate the amount of change they are supposed to receive after making a purchase.

Exercises in addition, subtraction, division, and other basic arithmetic skills, either with a therapist or as part of your home work with the survivor, can help stimulate the brain to relearn these skills. Computer programs are also available to assist with these problems (see Resource Guide).

Coping Strategies

If you know the survivor has problems with computation:

• Monitor all activities such as monetary transactions, measuring, and other forms of calculations.

• If he or she is taking medication, be sure to participate in counting the appropriate number of pills or measured doses of medicine. Then remove the remaining medication so that additional doses are not taken in error.

EFFECTS OF RIGHT-BRAIN INJURY ON COMMUNICATION

Damage to the right side of the brain may affect a person's nonverbal communication skills, including the ability to recognize facial expressions and the ability to assess appropriate communication behavior, such as the importance of taking turns in conversation or understanding the significance of tones of voice.

Pragmatic Deficit

Injury to the right side of the brain can produce pragmatic deficit, a situation in which the survivor fails to interpret nonverbal communication cues in conversations with others. Individuals with this condition usually have a good vocabulary and use correct grammar; however, they may talk too much or ramble, or they may say things that are completely off the topic under discussion.

If the person can write (if spatial-perceptual tasks are not a problem), he or she may write in a flowery way, using a lot of loops on letters and adding letters to words, such as "doog" or "appple."

Coping Strategies

As with other communication problems, pragmatic deficit often improves with time. In the interim you can help by using the following strategies:

• If the survivor rambles on and on, remind the person in an empathic, nonthreatening voice that others may wish to speak or that he or she must share the time.

• If speech becomes flowery, gently but firmly ask the person to come to the point.

• Steer the person back to the topic at hand whenever he or she goes off on a tangent.

GENERAL STRATEGIES FOR DEALING WITH COMMUNICATION PROBLEMS

Promoting effective communication with the stroke survivor will be made easier if you follow a few simple strategies:

• If the survivor wears dentures, make sure they fit correctly. This will facilitate speech for all survivors, especially those with dysarthria.

• Have the survivor's hearing checked to ensure there are no problems.

• Provide a positive environment that encourages the survivor to continue attempts to communicate. Accept and praise all efforts, both verbal and nonverbal. Encourage the survivor to combine verbal statements, whenever possible, with gestures such as pointing, nodding, and shaking the head yes or no.

• Establish eye contact with survivors when you communicate with them. This ensures that you have their attention, and they can watch your face and lips for clues that may improve understanding.

• Don't pretend you understand what the survivor is trying to say if you really don't. This will only create more confusion. Ask him or her to "say it another way," repeat, or use gestures. If you still can't understand, say, "Perhaps it's best if we come back to that later," and move on to something else.

• Don't address the survivor as if he or she is a child. Loss of the ability to communicate clearly does not mean the person is mentally or intellectually incompetent; even if a person cannot speak, he or she may still understand everything that is said.

• Give the survivor a little extra time to analyze what is heard or read. Speak slowly, to permit time to process what you have said.

• Wait patiently for a response. If you see he is struggling to respond, tactfully interpret what you think he is trying to say.

• Extra time is also needed when people with speech disorders switch from speaking to listening, or to writing. Again, you will need to be patient while the survivor processes thoughts or attempts to make a transition from one mode of communication to another.

• Resist the temptation to answer for the survivor in social situations. Don't try to "put words in her mouth" unless she is clearly struggling.

• Never talk about the survivor as if he weren't there. Even if he seems not to understand the content of the conversation, some comprehension may be taking place. What's more, body language, facial expressions, and the tone and volume of your voice all convey messages that may be understood.

• Always point out progress, and try to keep your expectations reasonable. Reaching one realistic goal, and receiving support for this achievement, will provide motivation to strive for the next goal.

ACTIVITIES TO IMPROVE COMMUNICATION SKILLS

Plan to spend some time each day on speech and language-skills activities. If you are already following a program developed in consultation with a speech-language pathologist or other professional, the following activities may supplement your current plan.

Choose a time when you're unlikely to be disturbed, and keep practice sessions to thirty minutes or less. If the survivor seems embarrassed doing these activities in the presence of others, wait until you are alone in the house. If the person becomes tired or frustrated, stop the session and start again later that day or the following day. These activities can be fun and are best approached in a lighthearted way:

• Label objects around the house using large block letters on white paper or cardboard. Ask the survivor to read the label and identify the object out loud. Cover one room at a time so that the survivor doesn't feel overwhelmed.

• Assemble a box of common household items, such as a spoon, fork, cup, toothbrush, pens, rubber bands. Ask the survivor to point to items as you name them. Or describe what each item is used for and ask him or her to point to the item you've identified.

• Bring out family albums and encourage the survivor to look at the pictures and identify the people in them. Talk about what is happening in each picture.

• Play games that promote practice with numbers, such as Twenty-one, solitaire, or dominoes.

• Encourage reading by cutting out bold headlines from magazines or newspapers.

• Take out large-print books from the library.

• Use word-search or picture-search puzzles to stimulate reading and speaking skills.

• Have the stroke survivor sing along with his or her favorite music.

• Try creative activities, such as painting, ceramics, photography, or sculpture, as alternative ways of communicating.

• Practice writing activities, such as copying shapes and letters. If possible, ask the survivor to help you write thank-you notes or postcards to friends.

Remember, relearning communication skills can be a frustrating, time-consuming process. If family members live nearby, ask them to help you with some of the communication activities, provided the survivor feels comfortable working with them.

Keep track of progress and achievements (see chapter 1, page 22). Acknowledge and reinforce every advance. Although much significant recovery usually occurs in the year following a stroke, gains can continue to be made for many years afterward.

FOUR

Helping with Physical Problems

I moved in with Dad shortly after he was discharged from the hospital. Although I tried to keep up a brave front, I felt devastated. Dad could barely put one foot in front of the other, and he had always been so strong! I took him to physical therapy every day for the first few weeks and also helped him practice at home. I'm ashamed to admit it, but a lot of the time I was furious. I blamed him—as though the stroke were his fault!—but I did the best I could to help.

Then, after about a month, he really did seem to be getting better. He was walking pretty well on his own, with a cane at first. I spoke with the physical therapist, who was very pleased with Dad's progress. So I felt more relaxed. Maybe he would fully recover, I thought. But whenever I remembered what he had been like—going to the gym, running, riding his bike—I felt depressed. . . .

Well, it's been six months since Dad had the stroke, and I have to admit I'm surprised. He walks a mile around the park every day, and he actually plans to start jogging next week! I never would have guessed it during those first weeks. I'm glad we both had staying power; in fact Dad probably had more motivation than I did!

—Gail

As we've seen, after a stroke even the most familiar and routine activities can be difficult for survivors. Getting out of bed and putting on a bathrobe becomes an ordeal. Cutting food or putting on a shirt with one hand is frustrating. Said one stroke survivor, "I knew where my mouth was, but my toothbrush couldn't find its way."

Caregivers play a crucial role in helping survivors regain their physical abilities, adapt to new ways of getting around, and take care of their own personal needs. Part of your role is also to ensure that the survivor is safe both at home and in the community as he or she makes these adjustments.

In this chapter we look at how you can help stroke survivors adjust to their physical limitations and become mobile again. Be aware that the return to mobility occurs in stages. At first you'll help the survivor by making sure he or she is properly positioned in a bed or chair and by helping with transfers (for example, from bed to wheelchair, or wheelchair to car seat). Then you will assist with the return to walking and other physical activities, such as dressing and bathing. You will learn some of the modifications you can make around the home and what aides are available to make the environment safe and "stroke-friendly."

VISION PROBLEMS

"I see the world in slices," said Ruth, who has *hemianopsia*—damage to the optic nerve, resulting in partial loss of vision. Hemianopsia may cause half vision in one or both eyes. As a result a male survivor may end up shaving only one side of his face; a female, applying lipstick to only one side of her mouth.

Hemianopsia may also cause a survivor to run a wheelchair into walls or doorways on the affected side, or he or she may not see someone sitting or standing on the affected side.

Unfortunately the problem is permanent, and cannot be corrected with surgery or glasses; however, the survivor can learn to compensate.

Visual acuity may also decrease after a stroke, preventing the survivor from seeing clearly.

Coping Strategies

If the survivor has vision problems after a stroke:

• Encourage the person to compensate by turning his or her head frequently in order to see an entire visual field.

• Encourage frequent scanning of the environment during all activities.

• Since eyes continue to adjust for up to six months following a stroke, do not buy new glasses or get a new prescription for the survivor during that time. Help the survivor to make do with the present set of glasses or to use a magnifying glass, if that is helpful, until the eyes have stabilized.

PARALYSIS

Many stroke survivors experience complete paralysis of one or more muscle groups after a stroke. Usually the side of the body opposite the side of the brain where injury occurs is most affected. For example left-brain injury may cause paralysis on the right side of the body, while right-brain injury may cause paralysis on the left side.

As a paralyzed limb goes through the process of recovering from a stroke, it generally follows a predictable sequence best described in terms of muscle tone. *Tone* is the readiness of muscle to contract on command from the brain.

The stages of recovery include the *flaccid stage,* which is characterized by absence of muscle tone (the affected limb feels limp, floppy, and possibly painful) and absence of reflexes and voluntary movement; the *beginning-spasticity stage,* in which muscle tone begins to come back, but there is no voluntary movement yet; the *full-spasticity stage,* which is characterized by excessive muscle tone and hyperactive reflexes (when you begin to bend or straighten one joint, the other joints in the same extremity bend or straighten too); and the *approaching-normal-tone stage,* in which spasticity decreases and the ability to move voluntarily increases, particularly the control over one joint.

Coping Strategies

Because the stages of recovery of movement may overlap considerably, certain techniques should be used daily in all stages:

• Full range-of-motion exercises should be performed, which include gently moving the survivor's head, arms, hands, legs, and feet at least once daily.

• Application of heat or electrical stimulation may be used to relieve painful joints.

• Stretching exercises can help relax spastic muscles and make joints more flexible.

• Spasticity can be "used" to help prepare the survivor for recovery. For example, the survivor can be encouraged to stand on a spastic limb in order to have the sensation of standing upright on both legs.

• Positioning of the body (described in the next section) should be done frequently.

Positioning

Proper positioning means ensuring that stroke survivors with some degree of paralysis sit, stand, and lie down in ways that keep their body in proper alignment. This will help prevent the development of crippling *contractures* (permanent shortening of muscles around a joint). If allowed to develop, muscle and joint contractures will limit the survivor's mobility indefinitely. Preventing them is a key to recovery.

Positioning is also vital for the prevention of *pressure sores,* or *bedsores,* ulcers that may form when blood pools in parts of the body as a result of immobility. Common sites are the shoulders, elbows, lower back, hips and buttocks, ankles and heels (see chapter 5 for details).

General Principles

Once you know the basic principles underlying the prevention of complications such as contractures and bedsores, you will be able to figure out when the survivor's body is in the correct position.

"I never realized how the body can shift out of shape when left to its own devices," Carol said. *"But repositioning Gary every time he would sit, stand, or lie down taught me not to take anything for granted. It was difficult; in fact in the first few days after he came home from the hospital, I felt almost obsessed with moving his arm into the 'right' place all the time.*

Fortunately by the end of the second week some voluntary movement returned, and Gary began to be able to move his arm into the right position by himself. But the whole experience was kind of spooky, as if the arm was this separate thing, not really attached to the rest of him. Sometimes I would get mad at the arm for being in the wrong place."

• Maintain normal anatomic alignment of the head, trunk, and limbs. For example, don't permit the survivor to sit on one hip or lean to one side persistently when sitting.

• Position each joint in the opposite direction from its spastic position as much as possible. For example, keep the fingers extended rather than curled closed, and maintain the ankle-foot angle at ninety degrees, rather than permitting the foot to remain extended forward.

• Help the survivor shift positions frequently in order to increase blood flow and help regain proper balance.

Supine Position

The survivor is properly positioned on his or her back when:

• The head is in midline position to normalize the tone of the trunk and limbs. Extend and align the neck with the back, using a pillow under the head to prevent flexion of the neck.

• The affected shoulder is in a forward position. Place a pillow under the affected arm and shoulder to keep the arm away from the body. The elbow should be slightly bent with the hand elevated.

• The trunk is fully extended with the spine in proper alignment.

• A folded towel is placed under the affected hip.

• A small rolled towel or pillow is placed along the outside of the affected leg (not under the knee) to keep it in proper alignment.

• The affected ankle is positioned at ninety degrees to prevent foot-drop. A foam wedge or high-top shoes can be used to support the foot.

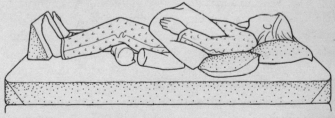

Supine position

Lying on the Affected Side

The survivor is properly positioned on the affected side when:

- The head is in midline position supported with a single pillow.
- The elbow of the affected arm is slightly bent and the shoulder is forward. A pillow may be placed under the unaffected arm.
- The trunk is fully extended and aligned. A pillow or wedge should be placed behind the back for support.
- The affected leg is nearly straight at the hip and slightly bent at the knee. The unaffected leg should be in a comfortable position for the survivor. A pillow should be placed between the legs.

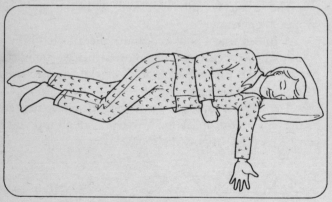

Lying on the affected side

Lying on the Unaffected Side

The survivor is properly positioned on the unaffected side when:

- The head is in midline position supported by a pillow.
- The affected arm is placed on a pillow with the

elbow as straight as possible. The hand should not hang over the edge of the pillow.

• The trunk is positioned with the affected side forward. A pillow or wedge should be placed behind the back.

• The affected leg is positioned with hip and knee slightly bent. A pillow should be placed lengthwise between the legs to support the foot, but the foot should not hang over the edge of the pillow.

• The unaffected leg is placed in a comfortable position.

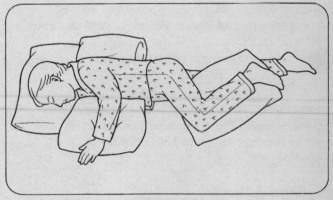

Lying on the unaffected side

Positioning Specific Body Parts

The following guidelines apply whether the survivor is sitting or standing:

• **Head and neck:** Head position affects the muscle tone of the trunk and limbs. If the head is always turned to one side, abnormal posture will develop, hindering mobility. When the survivor is standing, his or her head should be kept in a normal position, centered above the shoulders. In bed it is helpful to support the head with a pillow.

• **Trunk:** When sitting and standing, weight should be distributed as evenly as possible on both sides of the hips. If spasticity causes the survivor to lean more to one side when sitting, support the balanced position by using pillows or a foam wedge.

• **Shoulder:** Keep the upper arm and elbow out and away from the chest when the survivor is lying down.

• **Elbow:** Keep the elbow straight or slightly bent whenever possible.

• **Forearm and hand:** Position with the palm up, even when the hand is in the survivor's lap.

• **Wrist and fingers:** Extend the wrist backward and keep the fingers as straight as possible.

• **Hips, knees, and ankles:** Don't allow the limb to roll outward when sitting. The kneecap and toes should point straight ahead. Tuck a firm pillow or towel roll under the upper thigh to help keep the leg in the proper position.

Positioning Devices

Sometimes stroke survivors need a positioning device to counteract a spastic muscle or assist them until they regain muscle tone.

• **Slings:** Several types of slings may be used during various phases of recovery. A *hemi-sling* holds a flaccid arm and hand close to the body in order to prevent injury while the limb recovers tone. A *shoulder-girdle sling* allows the elbow and forearm to be free but holds the shoulder joint to prevent pain and maintain alignment while the muscles regain strength.

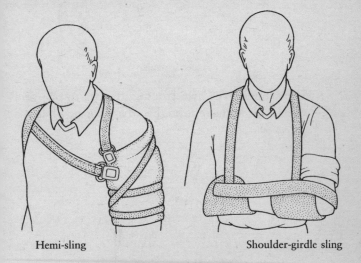

Hemi-sling   Shoulder-girdle sling

• **Resting-hand splint:** This device helps keep an affected hand in a functional position—wrist slightly extended, fingers open, and the thumb away from the palm.

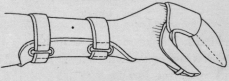

Resting-hand splint

• **Finger spreader:** A finger spreader keeps the affected hand relaxed with the fingers spread and the wrist slightly extended.

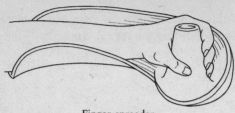

Finger spreader

• **Arm trough:** The arm trough attaches to one arm of a wheelchair and supports the affected arm while the survivor is seated.

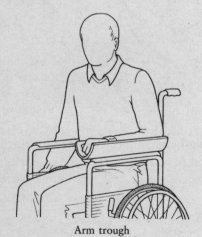

Arm trough

• **Lapboard:** Unlike the arm trough, this board lies across both arms of the wheelchair. It can also double as a work or eating surface.

"The lapboard really helps Dan," says his wife. "He lost part of his right visual field, but with the lapboard he can keep his affected arm in view, so he'll be reminded to use it as much as possible."

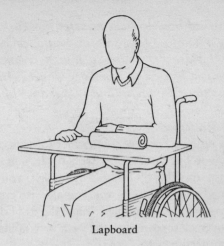

Lapboard

Transfers

Transfers involve moving the survivor from one seat to another, that is from wheelchair to commode or from wheelchair to car. There are two basic types of transfers: standing or sitting.

Survivors who are weak or paralyzed on one side may still be able to do a standing transfer provided they have adequate arm strength on the unaffected side and some degree of balance. Although you should be prepared to assist them, survivors should be encouraged to do as much of the transfer on their own as possible. The more they practice, the faster they'll improve.

Sitting transfers are used with survivors who are paralyzed in both legs or who for other reasons, such as severe weakness or illness, cannot help with a transfer.

Ethel learned how to help transfer her husband, Bob, by using a two-foot-long smooth board, called a sliding board. *"I place the board so that it creates a bridge from the seat he's on to wherever he needs to go. Then he moves onto the board and just slides," she says.*

Coping Strategies

When doing a transfer, remember to protect not only the survivor but yourself as well. Even if the survivor can do the transfer by himself or herself, you will need to be ready in the event the transfer isn't successful. This means you may suddenly have the full body weight of the survivor thrown against you, or you may have to catch the person before a fall:

• Always stand with your knees bent, with a feeling that your weight is centered in your lower body. If you are lifting or moving the survivor yourself, the major share of your work should be done by your quadriceps, the big muscles in the tops of your thighs, not your arms and upper or lower back.

• Prepare for the transfer. Talk to the survivor while moving him or her, saying what you are going to do before you do it and asking for the survivor's cooperation. If the survivor will do a standing transfer, talk about what he or she will do before actually attempting it. Shoes or braces should be on prior to initiating the transfer (unless of course the transfer is to the bathtub). A limp or paralyzed arm should be placed in a sling. If you need a sliding board, have it ready. If the transfer involves a wheelchair, make sure the brake is on, arm and foot rests are out of the way, and clothing is not caught on the chair.

• When possible, the surface you are transferring to and the one you are transferring from should be approximately the same height; alternatively the surface to which you are transferring the survivor should be lower than the starting point. It takes extra strength and practice to move from a lower to a higher level.

• Make sure the two surfaces are as close together as possible.

• In most cases survivors should lead with their stronger side during a transfer.

BECOMING MOBILE

One of the most important aspects of your role in recovery is to help the survivor become as mobile as possible. Achieving this goal may take time, patience, and perseverance on both your parts, but the results will be worth it.

The key to success in this process is to accept that recovering one's physical abilities occurs in stages. The person will progress over time from wheelchair dependence to the use of a walking aid such as a cane and then, one would hope, to independent walking. Your help and guidance are needed, literally, each step of the way. Although not every survivor will be capable of walking completely unaided, your primary concern should be to assist the person you're caring for to reach whatever level of physical independence he or she is capable of achieving.

Wheelchairs

Wheelchairs may be rented or purchased outright and come with an array of features that may help the survivor. Not every feature may be needed, however, so it's important to talk with the survivor's physical or occupational therapist before making any decisions.

Although a rental wheelchair may be adequate, many professionals believe that making the purchase is the best investment. It is difficult to assess whether a rental wheelchair is in good condition; also, even if a therapist projects that the survivor will need the chair on a temporary basis, no one can predict with accuracy how long the healing process will take. Finally, some survivors prefer to keep their wheelchairs for use in airports or at events that would require them otherwise to stand for extended periods of time, or if they feel they would have difficulty moving freely among large numbers of people.

Be sure to check with your insurance company to see whether the cost of a wheelchair is covered. Requirements vary from company to company.

Meanwhile some of the special features you might want to consider include:

• **Brake extension:** This detachable rod increases the leverage of the brake handle so that less strength is required to engage the brake.
• **Elevating foot and leg rests:** These are helpful for individuals who have swelling in the leg or foot.
• **Removable foot and leg rests:** This feature allows the survivor to begin to use his legs to help push and steer the wheelchair. During difficult transfers, remov-

able rests allow you to move the wheelchair in closer to the surface to which you are transferring the survivor.

• **Removable armrests:** Sliding transfers are easier if the armrests can be removed.

• **Wheelchair narrower:** When this device is turned, the sides of the wheelchair compress to allow the chair to go through an otherwise impassable doorway. This may cause some pressure on the survivor's hips, but it is only momentary. After it clears the doorway, the chair returns to its original width.

Wheelchair Ramps

Properly constructed ramps are an important asset if the survivor is wheelchair dependent for any length of time.

Tim's occupational therapist told us the best ramp for both pushing a wheelchair and self-wheeling should be built on a ratio of twelve inches of length per one inch of height. Our top step into the house is thirty inches high, so we needed a three-hundred-sixty-inch, or thirty-foot, ramp," said Leslie. After pricing commercial ramps, Leslie called her nephews. At a fraction of commercial prices they built a thirty-foot-long, four-foot-wide wooden ramp and covered it with indoor-outdoor carpeting.

Stroke survivors with two functioning arms or with a strong arm and a strong leg can usually self-wheel up a ramp with this grade. Although a person pushing a wheelchair can go up a steeper ramp, the above ratio should be followed for survivors who want to be self-wheeling.

Skills Needed to Resume Walking

Walking upright on both feet is a uniquely human ability, and one that every stroke survivor strives to regain. But because this ability is a highly developed and complex motor skill, certain requirements must be met before safe, functional walking is resumed:

• The survivor must have sufficient strength in at least one lower limb and in the trunk to compensate for stroke-related weakness.

• The stronger upper limb must have sufficient strength and coordination to hold on to and bear down on a cane or walker.

• A good sense of balance is vital. The survivor must be able to sit without back or arm support and stand on both feet without support. When they are seated, many stroke survivors overestimate their ability to balance themselves while standing.

• The amount of feeling survivors have on their affected side influences how well they can walk. They must have some ability to feel and touch and to know without looking what position their limbs are in.

• As noted earlier, good vision is critical for safe walking. People with hemianopsia can make adjustments for this visual problem as they relearn how to walk.

• Good spatial perception—knowing how far things are or where the body is in relation to other objects in the immediate environment—is essential. Knowing where our bodies are in space and the distance to objects around us are unconscious skills that can be disrupted by a stroke.

Walking Aids

"I don't need my cane. I'll just hold on to the furniture."

Despite what some stroke survivors say, furniture is not a walking aid. If they insist they can "furniture-walk" around the house, discourage them. Furniture comes in different heights, is not spaced evenly, and may move unexpectedly, causing the individual to fall.

An array of appropriate walking aids are available to help. Braces should be used during recovery to help the survivor reduce fatigue and avoid injury. As the survivor moves toward greater independence, the goal is to move from larger aids, such as a quad cane, to a smaller aid, such as a cane.

Braces

The purpose of a brace, also called an *orthosis,* is to compensate for weakness or problems in the muscles, bones, or joints. Although it can provide support for an activity such as walking, it cannot make a muscle stronger or improve the survivor's coordination.

Braces to support the foot and ankle, called an *ankle-foot orthosis,* or *AFO,* come in two basic types: (a) a metal device that attaches directly to the shoe and is worn under the pant leg; and (b) one made of lightweight plastic that is molded to the calf, ankle, and foot. The plastic version, which is sometimes referred to as a *leaf-spring brace*, fits inside the shoe and under the pant leg and can be used with different shoes. The metal braces must be used with the shoes to which they are attached.

Survivors who wear a brace need to be careful about the style of shoe they wear. If a metal brace is used, the shoe needs to have a steel shank. Oxford-style shoes are best for this purpose. People who wear a leaf-spring brace need to wear sturdy, enclosed shoes with flat soles.

Quads and Canes

Quad canes are canes with four small legs. These provide more support than an ordinary cane, promote balance, and help reduce fatigue. *Tripods,* which have three legs, should be avoided because they can cause a loss of balance.

Before progressing from a quad cane to a standard cane, the survivor should be able to stand alone without the cane and without someone supporting his or her arm or back.

To determine the correct cane height, measure the vertical distance from the crease in the survivor's wrist to the ground while the person is standing in walking shoes. This length should equal the distance from the tip of the cane to the top of the handle. If the cane is too long, the survivor will lean to the opposite side; if it is too short, he or she will lean forward and may fall.

The cane should have a rubber tip to prevent it from slipping. Check the tip frequently to make sure it has not worn through. For stroke survivors with arthritic hands, wrap the handle in foam rubber, available at many discount outlets and department stores.

When walking with an aid, stroke survivors should keep their elbows slightly bent. This prevents undue strain on the elbow and wrist joints. The walking aid should always be held by the stronger hand.

Talk with your physician or physical therapist to determine when it is appropriate for the survivor to move from one type of aid to another.

Walkers

Walkers (walking frames, walkerettes) have a major limitation: They encourage stop-and-start rather than normal walking. They also require the survivor to use two strong arms simultaneously, which can be a major problem.

ENVIRONMENTAL CHALLENGES

Of course becoming truly mobile, with or without an aid, generally involves more than simply moving back and forth on a level surface. Whether at home or out in the community, the environment poses challenges to everyone's sense of balance at times; these challenges can be especially daunting to the survivor, who may still be weak or trying to cope with a paralyzed limb. Following are some areas of special concern where your assistance may be needed.

Negotiating Steps and Stairs

If stairs are part of the stroke survivor's environment, railings should be placed on both sides of the stairs and a grab rail should be available at the top of the steps.

Take a good look at the steps the survivor will have to use. Ideally they will be no higher than six inches, a minimum of thirty inches wide, and a minimum of fourteen inches deep. Steps with these measurements will accommodate anyone who uses a quad cane. The surface of the steps should be flat and without cracks. If there is carpeting on the steps, be sure it is secure.

You can help stroke survivors maneuver up and down steps once you understand the sequence:

When going up, the survivor should:

1. Step up on the stair with the stronger leg while pushing down on the cane
2. Bring the affected leg up to the same step
3. Bring the cane up and repeat the process, stepping up first on the stronger leg, then bringing the affected leg to the same step

When going down, the survivor should:

1. Bring the cane down to the step surface
2. Bend the knee of the stronger leg to lower the body, but do not step down
3. Step down with the affected leg first, then with the stronger leg

Out and About

Venturing away from the home environment can bring some unexpected challenges for stroke survivors.

If the survivor is in a wheelchair, be aware that most public buildings, restaurants, malls, and businesses are wheelchair accessible and must have handicapped parking as required by law. However, don't assume compliance. If in doubt, call ahead. An old favorite restaurant may not accommodate wheelchairs, or it may have steps and no ramp.

If the survivor uses a cane or walker, be aware that it takes time to adjust to walking on sidewalks, grass, and in parking lots. Be prepared to assist the survivor the first few times he or she walks on these surfaces.

The survivor may be eligible for "handicapped" status for parking. Regulations vary from state to state. The first step is to contact your local motor vehicle department for appropriate application forms. In many states a physician fills out the form and the motor vehicle department then determines the survivor's eligibility.

Coping Strategies

When out and about, the survivor should:

- Be careful not to place a cane into cracks or lines in the cement
- Avoid puddles, gravel, mounds of dirt, or stones
- Take smaller steps when walking on inclines
- Move on and off curbs in the same way that he or she moves up and down steps
- See whether a device can be added to the tip of the

cane to provide more traction when walking in snow (see chapter 10)

PERFORMING OTHER DAILY ACTIVITIES

At the same time that they are learning to walk independently, survivors are also relearning basic physical skills, such as dressing and undressing and bathing themselves. You can help in these areas as well, by encouraging the survivor to do as much as possible on his or her own and at the same time by being available to help if needed.

Dressing and Undressing

Dressing and undressing can present big obstacles for survivors, especially if they don't have full use of their hands and fingers.

"I never thought I'd be dressing or undressing anyone again—much less my own husband," Clara said. *"But after the stroke, his body was totally paralyzed on the left side. He really couldn't do it himself. I admit it felt very strange to care for him like that, as though he were one of my children. I didn't like treating him that way, and I know he didn't like it either. But it had to be done."*

Coping Strategies

Although dressing and undressing can present a challenge for both the survivor and the caregiver, practicing the following techniques will make the process easier, until the survivor can take care of these needs as before. Also consider purchasing adaptive aids and clothing designed for people with physical limitations. Sources of these items are listed in the Resource Guide.

• The survivor should start by wearing loose clothing that closes in the front, and pants or skirts with elastic waistbands.

• Lay clothes out in the order in which they will be put on.

• Encourage the survivor to get dressed and undressed while sitting up rather than standing, especially at first. If the edge of a bed doesn't offer enough support, have him or her sit on a chair.

• Clothing should always be put on the affected arm or leg first. When undressing, the affected limb should be undressed first.

• Velcro fasteners may be used instead of buttons, especially in the early stages of relearning.

• Survivors can practice buttoning and unbuttoning clothes they are not wearing until they can master this task. A button hook may be helpful, especially in the first few months after the stroke. To help buttons stay aligned, clothing should be buttoned from the bottom up.

• Those with visual or perceptual difficulties may have trouble seeing buttons and buttonholes on clothes with bright prints or complex patterns. Solid colors and simple designs may be less confusing.

• Zippers are easier to pull up and down if a metal key-ring loop is attached to them. It also helps to button or snap pants or skirts before pulling the zipper up.

• Rather than a bulky coat for cold weather, try a

cape or poncho that goes over the head; instead of gloves, try mittens.

• When undressing, remember the general rule: What goes on last, comes off first.

Bathing

Like dressing and undressing, the ability to bathe oneself is something most of us take for granted. However, the survivor is not likely to be able to perform this task safely, especially in the first weeks after a stroke.

You may feel uncomfortable bathing the survivor, especially if you are a son or daughter—though even spouses may feel uncomfortable in this role. If you remind yourself that you are performing a vital job— keeping the survivor clean reduces the possibility of infection—the job may be somewhat easier. If you find that you really don't feel up to bathing the survivor, see whether you can hire a home health care worker to perform this and other personal-hygiene tasks (see chapter 1).

Coping Strategies

Even if the survivor can bathe himself or herself, you should monitor the person, either by staying in the room or by checking frequently. Making simple adaptations, such as those described below, are also helpful:

• Using a quad cane in the shower can help with balance and facilitates getting in and out of the shower or shower seat.

• If the survivor has lost sensation on one side and can't feel the water temperature, have him test it on his unaffected side, or test it for him. An unbreakable thermometer can also be placed in the tub.

• Shampoo bottles with flip tops are easier to open and close than those with screw-on tops.

• Thin cotton terry washcloths are easier to handle than thick ones.

• A long-handled brush can be used by survivors so that they can wash their backs, legs, and feet without having to reach around or bend down.

GUIDELINES FOR PREVENTING FALLS AND OTHER INJURIES IN THE HOME

Falls and injuries are always a danger during recovery, when the survivor is relearning so many activities. Chapter 10 contains resources for many different types of adaptive equipment that can be used around the house to facilitate the survivor's recovery and promote independence. You can make your home more "stroke-friendly" by using such devices as needed and following these steps:

• Remove throw rugs. Tack down the edges of carpets, especially where they end before going onto another surface.

• Secure all electrical and telephone cords or run them under the carpet.

• Are your doorways too narrow for a wheelchair? Individuals who use wheelchairs need at least thirty-two inches to push themselves through a doorway, twenty-nine inches if someone else pushes them through. To increase the width of door openings, you can remove the molding or the door.

• Move or rearrange any furniture that hinders walking or a wheelchair.

• Although most chair seats are fifteen inches high, it is easiest to get in and out of chairs with seats that are at least nineteen or twenty inches. You can raise the height of chair seats by placing double cushions on them. Placing wooden blocks under the chair legs is not recommended because they may throw the chair off balance.

• Have a light source near each doorway, or use night-lights.

• Keep a list of emergency telephone numbers next to each telephone.

A Room-by-Room Safety Guide

Kitchen

• Don't wax kitchen or bathroom floors.

• Have convenience appliances, such as a blender, electric can opener, electric skillet, and food processor, available if possible. This reduces the need for the survivor who wants to cook to use knives and other handheld tools that require fine-motor coordination skills.

• Use pots and pans with handles that don't conduct heat.

• Encourage the survivor to slide pots, plates, and pans along the countertop and stove rather than lift them.

- Use splatter screens on the stove.
- If the stove top is too hard to see or reach for individuals in a wheelchair, place a mirror over it so that they can see inside pots. If possible, use a hot plate, microwave, or toaster oven for cooking. These are safer than conventional range cooking.

Bathroom

- Install grab bars in and around the tub.
- Use a tub seat or bench in the shower or tub if the survivor has problems with balance, perception, or muscle weakness. The seat should be the same height as a wheelchair, approximately nineteen inches. Some tub seats have adjustable legs or back supports. If you cannot get a tub seat, place a sturdy nonrust chair that has rubber tips on the legs in the tub or shower stall.
- Place a rubber mat or decals on the tub floor to prevent slipping.
- Replace glass shower doors with a shower curtain.
- Most toilet seats are too low for survivors who use wheelchairs. Toilet guard rails or an elevated toilet seat can be installed to compensate.
- The ideal height for sinks for individuals who use wheelchairs is twenty-four inches from the floor. Place a regular chair under the sink if there isn't enough room for a wheelchair.
- Insulate exposed hot-water pipes under the sink to protect the survivor's legs while sitting.
- Faucets with a single horizontal lever can be pushed with the hand or wrist and may be easier for

stroke survivors to use than knobs that need to be turned.

Bedroom

• If your regular bedroom is on the second floor of the house, arrange a temporary one on the first floor until the survivor learns to go up and down stairs.

• The ideal height of the bed depends on the individual's limitations. Stroke survivors can sit down and get up from the edge of a high bed more easily than from a low one. However, if they have poor balance, a high bed allows their feet to dangle and makes it more difficult for them to feel stable while sitting. A low bed allows them to put their feet on the floor for stability, but individuals with a weak lower limb may find it hard to get up and sit down. Consult with a physical therapist to determine the best bed height for your situation.

• Make sure the bed is stable, preferably up against a wall. If you are using a hospital bed, lock the brakes.

• Clothes should be hung on rods that are thirty-six inches from the floor for easy accessibility to survivors in wheelchairs. Shoes and accessories can be placed in shoe bags that hang from the door.

• Place a telephone or emergency buzzer within easy reach of the bed.

As the survivor becomes mobile and begins once again to resume daily activities, the activity-and-progress log described in chapter 1 takes on increasing importance for both you and the survivor. Charting progress will enable you to stay motivated and have a sense of accomplishment. Although it won't totally make up for the physically and emotionally exhausting days, and the adaptations you may have to make to your home, it can certainly give you a boost to realize how far along you've both moved on the road to stroke recovery!

FIVE

Your Role in Medical Therapy

I was used to Mary's taking insulin because she's had diabetes for years. But when she came back from the hospital after the stroke, she had half a dozen different pills to take as well. It was so complicated—diuretics for blood pressure, an antidepressant for her moods. Even the amount of insulin she had to take was changed.

It was hard to keep them all straight, so I made a chart and color-coded the bottles. The doctor told me to watch for side effects, but how could I tell? Sometimes she acted strange from the stroke; I couldn't separate the symptoms from the medication. Even getting her to the doctor was difficult.

After the first couple of weeks I knew I needed help. So I got a part-time health care worker and she took care of the medications and lots of other things. That made caring for Mary a lot easier.

—Frank

Numerous medical problems may emerge after a person has sustained a stroke. In addition to complications from the stroke itself—which may include among others swelling; pressure sores; seizures; blood clots; gastrointestinal, musculoskeletal, respiratory, and emotional problems—the survivor may have preexisting conditions such as high blood pressure, diabetes, or arthritis that also require treatment.

This situation has several implications for caregivers. First it is important to make sure one physician is in charge of coordinating the survivor's care and monitoring his or her medical problems. In addition, if possible, one pharmacist should be selected to supply needed medications, explain how and when they should be administered, and help avoid drug-drug interactions. Finally, you will need to become familiar with the survivor's medical problems and medications, coordinate pill-taking regimens, and keep an eye out for signs of drug side effects or symptoms that indicate a given disorder may be worsening and require immediate professional attention.

Although so much responsibility may seem daunting, this chapter can help. We'll provide tips on how to select a coordinating physician and pharmacist as well as other health professionals and how to manage medications. Plus we'll take an in-depth look at the complications of stroke and their treatment.

SELECTING A PHYSICIAN TO COORDINATE CARE

Ideally the person coordinating the survivor's medical care would be your present physician—a general practitioner or internist who knows the survivor's medical history and prestroke personality.

However, it's possible that you don't have such a doctor now. Although many families used to have a family physician who followed them over many years, the dramatic changes that have taken place in our health care system in recent years have changed this situation for many people.

Today you may belong to a managed-care system or have a health care plan that permits you to choose from among a small pool of member physicians rather than selecting from among all physicians. If this is the case for you, then your choices may be limited. Nevertheless most health care plans do permit you at least some choice. So if you don't feel comfortable with your present physician, you should exercise your right to make other choices.

When seeking a new physician, compile a list of doctors whose work is praised by people you respect—friends, family members, community leaders, other health care workers, other physician specialists. You may also consult the *Dictionary of Medical Specialists,* which is available at your local library.

Next set up consultation appointments with each prospective physician. Be prepared to pay a fee, usually equal to the fee of a standard office visit. When setting the consultation appointment, get as much information as you can about how the doctor runs the practice, including office hours, waiting time for appointments, and payment schedule. In addition to eliciting helpful information, asking questions permits you to assess the cordiality and professionalism of the office staff.

Following are some tips for finding the best possible physician to coordinate the survivor's care and be available to respond to your questions and concerns. When you have narrowed your selection to one or two physicians, consider bringing the survivor with you to an interview to see how they interact.

What to Look for in a Physician: A Checklist

A good physician provides you with information in a forthright way, treats you with respect and concern, and has an office staff that is efficient and friendly. It's best to "doctor-shop" as early in the rehabilitation process as possible, but it's never too late to change if you feel your current physician is not meeting your needs. This checklist provides you with questions to ask yourself during the selection process:

Does the doctor

_____communicate with me in a way I can understand without being condescending? Allow me to express fears about the survivor's symptoms or certain forms of treatment? Give me real information about the survivor's condition instead of a simple pat on the back and reassurance?

_____seem knowledgeable about stroke, including the latest treatment options and strategies to prevent a second stroke?

_____explain medical tests and procedures before performing them? Discuss potential side effects or complications?

_____take time to answer my and the survivor's questions without rushing us?

_____talk with the survivor as a person before beginning an examination? Treat us courteously and with respect?

_____behave in an authoritarian way? Or in an easygoing manner?

_____seem comfortable with the idea of my getting a second opinion? Or threatened and defensive?

_____have a staff that is efficient and friendly?

_____have regular office hours during the day, evenings, and on weekends? Have a backup physician when he or she is not available?

_____regularly keep to the appointment schedule instead of keeping us waiting for long periods in the waiting room?

_____permit me to pay over time when visits aren't covered by insurance?

_____permit me to pay by check or credit card?

SELECTING OTHER HEALTH PROFESSIONALS

As we saw in chapter 1, you are likely to be part of a stroke-recovery team that may include such health care professionals as a neurologist; physiatrist; or speech, physical, and occupational therapists. You may stay in contact with the professionals who worked with the survivor in the hospital, or you may need to select appropriate specialists now, to assist in the rehabilitation process.

The same criteria described above may be used to select other health professionals. However, it is particularly important that the survivor feel comfortable with a specialist, especially if he or she will see the person on a regular basis. If possible, bring the survivor with you to the interviews and permit him or her to become involved in the selection process.

Selecting a Pharmacist

A pharmacist, like any other health professional, should be chosen with care. Registered pharmacists have special training and education in pharmaceuticals —prescription and over-the-counter drugs. As noted earlier, they are often in the best position to talk about potential side effects of medication, possible interactions among various medicines the survivor may be taking, how often to take a particular medicine, whether to have it before or with meals, and any other issues pertaining to the medicines the survivor may be taking for stroke-related problems and other medical conditions. Although these concerns should also be discussed with a physician, a physician may not be aware of all aspects of importance for each and every medication. That is the responsibility of the pharmacist.

Like a good physician, a good pharmacist should be willing to respond to your questions and concerns. The pharmacist can also act as a medication coordinator, staying alert to possible adverse interactions, expired prescriptions, and so on. Many pharmacies today have computerized records for each customer, noting all the medications they are taking (assuming of course that you purchase them in the same pharmacy). Some also have computer software that automatically alerts them to potential drug interactions when an additional medicine is prescribed.

If the survivor has chronic conditions that require

treatment over long periods of time, it's in the best interests of both of you to make friends with a pharmacist and take advantage of his or her specialized knowledge. The way to tell whether a pharmacist will be responsive to your needs is to ask questions and gauge his or her willingness to respond candidly and helpfully.

Of course cost of medication is also an important factor. You probably won't want to patronize a pharmacy that consistently offers products at higher prices than other nearby pharmacies. However, once you establish a relationship with a pharmacist where medications are competitively priced, if you happen to see a product advertised for less at a competing pharmacy, you may ask if your pharmacist will meet that price.

LIFESTYLE CHANGES BEFORE DRUG THERAPY

In this chapter we will emphasize the importance of medication in treating some of the complications that can follow a stroke, as well as some preexisting medical conditions. However, in many cases lifestyle changes should be tried before medication when possible. For example, proper diet and regular exercise, as well as quitting smoking, can help lower blood pressure, reduce gastrointestinal problems, and limit the need for medication.

Stress-reduction techniques such as visualization and meditation can be helpful in reducing the tension and anxiety that may lead to inappropriate behaviors or depression. In some cases they may also reduce pain by helping the survivor to relax. Stretching and range-of-motion exercises, described in chapter 4, can also help reduce pain in muscles and joints.

Of course other conditions, such as edema (swelling), blood clots, and seizures, will require medication. Medication will also be necessary if lifestyle changes are not effective enough, or if the survivor is not ready to implement them; for example if the survivor has very limited mobility, it won't be possible to attain the level of exercise required to lower blood pressure, or if the survivor has chewing and swallowing problems, then foods high in fiber can't be incorporated into the diet as easily.

DRUGS: WHAT EVERY CAREGIVER SHOULD KNOW

As a caregiver you have the responsibility of watching for and reporting to the physician any side effects, behavior changes, and symptoms that could be associated with the survivor's medications. Being alert to side effects is particularly important when the survivor has difficulty communicating and may not be able to let you know how he or she is feeling. Of course if the survivor can't read or is confused, you alone may be responsible for ensuring that the correct medications are taken, in the proper doses.

To become as informed as possible about each medication, ask your physician or pharmacist the following questions. To ensure that you remember all responses, take notes, ask for written instructions, or tape your conversation.

- What is this drug supposed to do for the problem?
- What are the side effects, both common and infrequent?
- What time(s) of day should the drug be taken?
- Should the drug be taken with food, before or after meals, or on an empty stomach?
- Should certain foods be avoided while taking this medicine?
- Is the drug available in another form? If it's a tablet, can it be ground up and mixed with food? Survivors who have trouble swallowing may find it easier to take a ground-up pill mixed with applesauce, or a liquid form if available.
- Should certain activities be avoided while taking this medicine?
- How long should the medication be taken?
- How long until some benefit will be apparent?
- Might it interact with other drugs the survivor is taking?

Organizing Medicines

"Victor is taking four different medications," says his wife, Gretchen. "Keeping them all straight—correct dosages, when to give them, and special instructions—is confusing. I need an easy and accurate way of handling it."

Gretchen's problem may be solved by using a basic chart that has the following columns:

NAME OF MEDICATION:
PRESCRIBED TO TREAT:
PRESCRIBING PHYSICIAN:
STARTING DATE:
LOOKS LIKE (e.g., pink tablet, white capsule)
WHEN TO TAKE:
HOW TO TAKE:
PURCHASED AT:
MAY RENEW:

Consider drawing the chart on a large, washable memo board so that you can make changes easily. Keep an extra copy on paper with you for when you visit the doctor.

For survivors who have difficulty seeing or who are only mildly confused, develop a color-coded system. Next to the name of each medication place a large colored sticker that matches one that you place on each dispensing container.

Pills can also be placed in morning, noon, dinner, and bedtime sections to correspond to the time that the pill should be taken. The containers can be filled by the caregiver to be sure the correct dosage is taken at the correct times.

TREATING COMPLICATIONS OF STROKE

On the following pages we will review the treatment of common complications of stroke as well as preexisting conditions that may require continued medication. Each section explains the problem, the types of medication used in treatment, and potential benefits and side effects. Use it as a handy reference if you suspect a problem or a worsening of the survivor's condition, in which case you should contact your physician immediately.

Edema

Edema is swelling of the feet, legs, or other body parts due to poor positioning, decreased blood circulation, general lack of mobility, kidney or bladder disturbances, or diabetes.

Diuretics are commonly prescribed for this condition. These agents decrease excess fluid in the body by increasing urine output.

Commonly prescribed diuretics include, among others, Midamor, Bumex, and Lasix. These drugs may cause the following side effects:

- Fall in blood pressure
- Rash
- Photosensitivity—when the skin becomes abnormally sensitive to sunlight, and brief exposure can cause rashes
- Nausea and vomiting
- Headache
- Dizziness or fainting
- Leg cramps
- Dehydration and electrolyte imbalances
- Increased blood sugar

Along with drug treatment edema may be treated by elevating the swollen limb above the heart level and increasing the amount of movement in general, including the range of motion and strength exercises prescribed by the physical and occupational therapists. If swelling persists, the physician may suggest using a pressure garment, which is worn on the affected limb until swelling subsides.

Pressure Sores

Pressure sores, or bedsores, are ulcers that develop on the skin of people who are bedridden, unconscious, or immobile for extended periods.

"I always associated pressure sores with people who were bedridden," said Stanley. "My wife's in a wheelchair, so when she got a bad sore on her left buttock, I was surprised. Yet I remember the nurse telling me to watch for them."

The sores start as red, painful areas that become purple before the skin breaks down, developing into open sores. Once the skin is broken, they may become infected, large, and slow to heal. Pressure sores should be checked out by a nurse or physician. Bedsores that are not infected can be treated with dressings, creams, or powders. If infection sets in, antibiotics may be prescribed.

Seizures

From five to ten percent of survivors may experience seizures—sudden episodes of uncontrolled electrical activity in the brain that may cause tingling or twitching of an area of the body, hallucinations, fear, or other intense feelings—following stroke. Sometimes a seizure is little more than a tingling or twitching in a small area of the body, such as a leg or an arm. In such cases notify your physician immediately after the seizure has passed.

Grand mal seizures, in which the person loses consciousness, and arms, legs, and head may twitch uncontrollably, are uncommon after stroke unless the person has a prior history of epilepsy or the seizure is a reaction to medication.

If the survivor does experience a seizure, move objects that may harm the person out of the way. Contrary to popular belief, biting the tongue is rare during a seizure; no attempt should be made to prevent it by wedging the mouth open. Once the seizure is over, call your physician or 911.

If the possibility of recurrent seizures exists, an anticonvulsant such as Dilantin or Tegretol may be prescribed. Side effects from such medications may include the following:

- Nausea and vomiting
- Diarrhea or constipation
- Lethargy
- Depression
- Confusion
- Sedation
- Headache
- Gait disturbance (problems walking)
- Slurred speech
- Tremors
- Dizziness
- Photosensitivity (sensitivity to light)

Blood Clots and Deep-Vein Thrombosis

The formation of blood clots in the thigh or calf, often called deep-vein thrombosis, occurs in more than fifty percent of stroke survivors. A clot, or thrombus, may form whenever the flow of blood in the arteries or veins is impeded. The risk is high among survivors because they are usually immobile and have a paralyzed limb; thus blood does not circulate well through the body, especially through the legs.

In some cases a pulmonary embolism (a blood clot that breaks away from the blood vessel and travels to the lungs) develops, which can cause lung damage, cardiac arrhythmias, and sudden death.

The following symptoms may indicate the presence of blood clots; if you notice any of them in the survivor, contact your physician:

- Leg pain
- Red areas on the calf
- Warm spots on an extremity
- Blood pressure fluctuations
- Shortness of breath
- Chest pain
- Swelling

Blood clots are preventable and treatable. As a preventive measure the anticoagulant heparin may be given for two to three months following a stroke. Anticoagulants increase blood-clotting time, thus permitting blood to flow more freely through the body—by decreasing the number of blood-clotting factors that are produced by the liver.

Depending on the results of a physical examination, the physician will prescribe drugs that either decrease blood clotting (anticoagulants such as heparin or Coumadin) or help dissolve existing clots (antiplatelets, such as aspirin). Anticoagulants and aspirin should not be taken at the same time. Also tell your physician about any cuts, falls, or burns, since an anticoagulant may prevent blood from clotting sufficiently for wounds to heal.

Following are anticoagulant side effects you should look for and report:

- Sudden bleeding
- Blood in the urine or stool
- Areas that bruise easily
- Bleeding gums
- Rash
- Fever
- Nausea and vomiting
- Fever

Antiplatelet drugs may also cause side effects, including:

- Gastrointestinal irritation
- Nausea
- Heartburn
- Ringing in the ears
- Flushing
- Anemia
- Bruising
- Ulceration and bleeding

Musculoskeletal Complications

Loss of muscle tone (flaccidity) and sensation, the development of spasticity (increased rigidity in a group of muscles, causing stiffness and restriction of movement), and trauma to the affected side of the body make stroke survivors prone to musculoskeletal complications.

"My father slid off the side of the bed while he was sitting down," said Kathleen. "He seemed to be all right, but the next day the arm on his affected side was swollen and discolored. We called the doctor right away."

In addition to swelling and skin discoloration, pain in the extremities, changes in mobility of limbs or joints, and any injury such as Kathleen's father experienced should be reported to the physician.

Spasticity

Treatment of spasticity can reduce or eliminate the risk of musculoskeletal problems. In many stroke survivors repetitive muscle-stretching exercises and proper positioning techniques (see chapter 4) will help correct this condition. Ice massage or heat packs may offer short-term relief.

Drug treatment includes the use of skeletal-muscle relaxants such as Baclofen or Valium. Such drugs can cause drowsiness and muscle weakness. Baclofen may also cause nausea and dizziness.

Anesthetic techniques such as motor point or nerve blocks may be prescribed for persistent spasticity. These involve injecting alcohol or phenol into the affected nerves. Treatment lasts for two to six months, allowing time for the muscle to recover.

Shoulder-Hand Syndrome

A condition called *reflex sympathetic dystrophy* involves pain, swelling, and problems controlling the movement of the upper and lower limbs. Called *shoulder-hand syndrome* when it affects those body parts, the condition sometimes occurs between the second and fourth months following a stroke.

"After two months of therapy Bill's hand swelled and was tender, and his shoulder hurt whenever he did his range-of-motion exercises," said his wife. "He wanted to quit therapy. But the doctor gave him some medication so that he would keep up the passive stretching and strengthening exercises."

An antidepressant such as amitriptyline or steroids such as prednisone may be used to treat pain in survivors with this condition. (For possible side effects of antidepressants, see the section on treating behavioral changes, page 121; steroids must be carefully managed to avoid blood problems.) Side effects may include weight gain, muscle weakness, and a range of systemic problems, including hypertension and gastrointestinal disorders.

Respiratory Complications

Survivors who have difficulty chewing and swallowing (see chapter 6) may develop *aspiration pneumonia*. This occurs when food or fluid gets into an unprotected airway. Although most people react by choking and coughing, some may aspirate (suck into the airway) without showing these symptoms. Report any of the following to your physician:

- Coughing or choking
- Difficulty swallowing
- Shortness of breath
- Noisy or raspy breathing
- Sudden changes in mental status
- Fever

In some cases the first symptom of aspiration pneumonia may be a high fever, which means infection is likely to have set in. In this case the survivor will be treated with antibiotics. If infection has not yet set in but the respiratory system is inflamed, then anti-inflammatory medications will be prescribed.

Gastrointestinal Complications

A stroke often disrupts eating habits and reduces appetite. These problems, along with lack of mobility, the intake of different drugs, and stress can lead to gastrointestinal upset, bleeding, or constipation. Contact your physician if the survivor has any of the following symptoms of gastrointestinal complications:

- Black or tarry stools
- Hard stools or loose, watery diarrhea
- Bloated stomach
- Reduced frequency or quantity of bowel movements

- Stomach pain
- Bloody vomit

Treatment will depend on the type of problem diagnosed, which may range from ulcers to simple constipation. Reviewing treatment of all potential gastrointestinal problems is beyond the scope of this book. However, because constipation is such a common problem, it is addressed in the following section.

Constipation

"Nearly everyone in my stroke-caregiver's group says the same thing—his or her spouse or parent gets recurrent constipation. Isn't there any way of preventing it?"

Recurrent constipation is frequently a result of lack of activity, insufficient fluids or dietary fiber, or the side effects of medication. First try increasing liquids (drink six to eight glasses of water or noncaffeinated beverage a day) and dietary fiber (fruits, vegetables, and whole grains, especially bran products).

If the above strategies aren't effective, your physician may suggest giving soap-solution enemas, temporarily using suppositories, or prescribing a stool softener or bulk agent. Oral laxatives are avoided because they may trigger an acute reaction or cause dependence, thus increasing constipation. If bleeding, abdominal pain, or bloating occur during such a program, contact your physician.

Regardless of the approach used, always ensure that the survivor has adequate privacy and sufficient time to sit on the toilet or commode chair.

Urinary Tract Infections

Urinary problems can result from inadequate fluid intake, infection, loss of sensation, or medications. Report any of the following observations to the physician:

- Urinary incontinence or retention
- Change in the frequency of voiding
- Painful urination
- Changes in color (bloody, brown), odor, or consistency of urine

Treatment of urinary tract infection varies depending on the cause of the infection. Antibiotics may be prescribed.

Urinary Incontinence

"The doctor told me most stroke survivors eventually get back control of their bladder," said Peter. "Boy, that was a relief to me! We had a terrible time those first few weeks after Maria came home from the hospital. She never seemed to be able to get to the bathroom fast enough. Sometimes she didn't even feel the urge to go, but there it was! I felt very uncomfortable treating her like a baby, and she was embarrassed too. Thank goodness everything's back to normal again."

Bladder function is often affected after a stroke. Although some survivors have trouble passing urine (retention), incontinence (the inability to control the passing of urine) is a more common problem. Attempts to reestablish normal bladder function begin in the hospital and may continue once the survivor returns home.

Maria, like most stroke survivors who have had urinary incontinence, had to relearn the voiding process. Following are ways of dealing with this problem:

• Tell the survivor to signal for assistance when the urge is felt. Those confined to bed or using wheelchairs may need help in using a bedside commode or getting to the bathroom.

• Suggest that the survivor go to the bathroom every two hours during waking hours to prevent the bladder from filling up. To stimulate the bladder, he or she can gently tap the lower abdomen. Some say the sound of running water helps. One woman even played a tape of ocean waves to encourage herself to urinate!

• Restrict fluids after the evening meal and encourage voiding prior to bedtime. If incontinence persists, monitor liquid intake. Survivors should drink at least one to one and a half quarts daily at regular intervals and avoid alcohol and coffee, which prompt urination.

• Kegel exercises—specific exercises to strengthen the pelvic and vaginal muscles—should also be practiced. These exercises, which involve stopping the flow of urine by contracting the muscles five or six times during voiding, can be taught by a physician or physical therapist. The exercises are usually performed on arising and during each voiding until control is relearned.

Some survivors have persistent incontinence despite retraining efforts. For men, an external condom catheter may be prescribed. These catheters attach to a leg bag for day use and a bed bag for nighttime. The catheter should be changed every day and the skin washed and dried carefully.

Women with persistent incontinence can use disposable adult diapers or waterproof underpants. Thorough daily cleaning and skin lubrication is essential when using these garments.

Survivors who use catheters or disposable waterproof undergarments may develop a urinary tract infection. Watch for the symptoms described in the section above as well as the following:

• Foul-smelling or cloudy urine with sediment
• Pain in the lower back
• Burning feeling around the catheter or when urinating
• Cramps in the lower abdomen or side
• Chills and fever
• Blood in the urine
• Frequent voiding
• An intense, frequent urge to urinate

Contact your physician immediately if these symptoms occur.

Pain

Two classes of medicines are generally prescribed to treat pain associated with stroke. These are narcotic analgesics, used prior to painful situations such as physical therapy, and nonsteroidal anti-inflammatory drugs (NSAIDs), which may be used to reduce inflammation in muscles and joints and treat headache and other types of pain.

Narcotic Analgesics

"The doctor told my husband to take his pain medication before he goes to physical therapy. Why is that?"

Drugs that are derived from morphine, such as codeine, hydrocodone, propoxyphene, and oxycodone, work best when they are given before physical therapy begins so that the survivor may complete therapy sessions with as little pain as possible. If the side effects of these drugs are troublesome, talk with your doctor to see whether NSAIDs can be taken instead of narcotic analgesics.

To prevent the nausea, vomiting, and gastric upset narcotic analgesics may cause, they should be taken with food or milk. Other possible side effects may include the following:

- Dizziness
- Drowsiness and fatigue
- Constipation
- Tremors
- Shortness of breath
- Restlessness
- Euphoric mood

Nonsteroidal Anti-inflammatory Drugs (NSAIDs)

Like narcotics, NSAIDs should be taken with food or milk to reduce the possibility of side effects. However, they should not be taken by anyone who is also taking aspirin. Common NSAIDs include ibuprofen, Voltaren, Indocin, and Clinoril.

Possible side effects include the following:

- Loss of appetite
- Bloating
- Headache
- Fatigue
- Depression
- Confusion
- Itching
- Chest pain
- Blurred vision
- Constipation

Behavior Problems and Depression

"Everyone was very patient with my father," says Doreen. *"But he refused to cooperate with the speech therapist or the physical therapist. He was disoriented, and none of our attempts to motivate him in rehab seemed to help."*

Survivors who are disoriented or uncooperative may be reacting to the sudden loss of function, self-esteem, independence, communication skills, and other limitations resulting from the stroke.

If these behaviors persist after members of the rehabilitation team have tried different behavioral- and communication-management techniques, such as those suggested in chapters 2 and 3, or if the behaviors are severe enough to make the survivor a danger to himself or herself or to others, then your physician may refer the survivor to a psychologist or a psychiatrist for consultation and/or treatment with medication.

Three classes of drugs are generally used: (a) antianxiety agents or (b) antidepressants may be prescribed to help relieve depression, or antipsychotic agents may be prescribed to help control severe behavior problems, such as aggression and agitation.

Antianxiety Agents

Stroke survivors who are given antianxiety agents, such as Xanax, Librium, or Tranxene, need to be monitored closely. Sometimes an antianxiety drug has unexpected results, as Lorraine discovered:

"After several months of therapy, Morris was highly agitated and often so confused, I got scared. The psychiatrist prescribed medication, but instead of their making him better, he got worse! Isn't an antianxiety drug supposed to make people less anxious?"

It is not unusual for an antianxiety drug to increase the level of agitation and confusion, especially among elderly individuals. Often a change to another drug will eliminate the problem, as it did in Morris's case. In addition to an increase in anxiety symptoms, look for the following side effects in individuals taking antianxiety drugs:

- Drowsiness and fatigue
- Poor voluntary muscle movement (ataxia) that was not evident before taking the drug

- Involuntary twitches of the face, trunk, or extremities
- Dizziness or fainting
- Nausea
- Constipation
- Rash
- Headache
- Urinary retention
- Weight gain or loss
- Vivid dreams or hallucinations
- Depression
- Restlessness

Antidepressants

In chapter 2, we discussed the signs of depression. Depression can be treated with psychotherapy, drugs, or both, depending on the needs of the stroke survivor. Some common antidepressants include Elavil, Asendin, and Prozac.

Antidepressants can cause many of the same side effects seen with antianxiety drugs. Some additional adverse effects include the following:

- Low blood pressure
- Blurred vision
- Uncontrolled lip smacking, chewing, or tongue movements
- Rigidity
- Parkinson's syndrome with tremor
- Dysphagia (difficulty in swallowing not associated with the stroke)
- Photosensitivity

Antipsychotic Agents

Antipsychotic agents, such as alprazolam and chlordiazepoxide, are used to control severe behavior problems such as aggression and agitation. Possible side effects include the following:

- Sedation
- Dry mouth
- Blurred vision
- Rapid heart rate
- Constipation
- Confusion
- Nightmares
- Parkinson's syndrome with tremor
- Changes in appetite and weight
- Lip smacking, uncontrolled chewing or tongue movements, involuntary twitches

Hypertension

Untreated high blood pressure is a major cause of stroke—and of a second stroke (see chapter 9). More than 80 percent of acute-stroke patients are hypertensive when they are admitted to the hospital. In some cases a stroke can initiate hypertension in a person who did not have high blood pressure before the stroke.

Control of hypertension for most stroke survivors includes proper diet and weight control (see chapter 6), exercise, stress reduction, and—if needed in addition to these strategies—medication.

Here we look at the different classes of drugs used to treat hypertension. Diuretics, which are discussed in the section on edema (page 108), may also be prescribed for hypertension. Other drugs include *beta-blockers, calcium channel blockers,* and *ACE inhibitors.*

Beta-blockers

Beta-blockers such as Sectral, Tenormin, and Inderal are used to lower blood pressure, as well as to treat heart disease. They may be prescribed along with a low-dose diuretic. Side effects may include:

- Fatigue
- Dizziness
- Confusion
- Depression
- Nausea
- Diarrhea
- Edema

If the person you are caring for has any of these symptoms and decides he or she wants to stop taking the drug, contact your physician immediately. Beta-blockers should not be stopped suddenly. The physician will explain how to cut the dosage gradually.

Calcium Channel Blockers

Calcium channel blockers, such as Cardizem and Cardene, are members of another class of drugs that help lower blood pressure. Possible side effects of these drugs include:

- Dizziness
- Headache
- Constipation
- Edema

- Rash
- Change in heart rate or rhythm

ACE Inhibitors

Angiotensin-converting enzyme (ACE) inhibitors, yet another group of medications to lower blood pressure, include drugs such as Capoten, Vasotec, and Prinivil.

These drugs are sometimes given to individuals who have both hypertension and diabetes, but they are usually avoided for people with kidney disease.

Side effects may include:

- Rash
- Dizziness
- Change in heart rate
- Chest pain
- Headache
- Hacking cough
- Metallic taste

Diabetes

According to the National Survey on Stroke, more than 20 percent of stroke survivors have diabetes. People with diabetes have difficulty metabolizing fat, and over time poor fat metabolism may lead to atherosclerosis, or hardening of the arteries in the heart, brain, and elsewhere in the body. Atherosclerosis is a major risk factor for stroke since it leads to poor circulation of blood. Therefore people with diabetes are at increased risk of having a stroke.

After a stroke the severity of diabetes changes in some individuals. Your physician should monitor blood glucose levels to determine whether the survivor's diabetes status has been altered.

Survivors with diabetes also need to be aware of poor circulation in their feet and legs, particularly on their affected side. The soles of the feet should be checked several times daily for bruises, cuts, and hangnails. Corns and calluses should be treated by a physician. Tight shoes, socks, or stockings with elastic can further reduce circulation and should be avoided. If you don't already have a podiatrist (specialist in foot problems) as part of your rehabilitation team, consider consulting with one.

To help maintain healthy feet in diabetic stroke survivors, do the following:

• Wash the feet in warm, not hot or cold, water. Do not use soaps that contain fragrance or deodorant.

• Massage the feet using a lanolin-base cream or lotion once or twice a day.

• Dry the feet thoroughly and remove any extra cream. Keep the skin between the toes dry with talcum powder.

Administering Insulin and Monitoring Sugar Levels

"After Troy's stroke, I had to learn how to give his daily insulin injections and watch his blood sugar levels," says Edie. "A counselor from the American Diabetes Association showed me how to use the self-monitoring blood sugar meters and how to use the needles. Eventually Troy gained strength and flexibility, and they helped him relearn how to do it."

If a counselor is not available, a nurse or physician can teach you the proper techniques for giving injections and monitoring blood sugar.

Some stroke survivors with diabetes may require oral hypoglycemic pills. If you are caring for someone who takes this medication, alert your physician if he or she is also taking any of the following drugs, which can cause variations in blood sugar levels: aspirin, diuretics, estrogen, niacin, adrenaline, decongestants that contain epinephrine or ephedrine, cough remedies, nasal sprays that contain phenylephrine, or over-the-counter drugs that contain caffeine.

Survivors with diabetes usually follow the same dietary plan they had before the stroke. However, if eating problems are preventing them from following their previous diabetic diet, consult with your physician or dietitian.

Dental Care

"After the stroke, Josh's dentures kept slipping. They didn't fit right anymore," says his wife, Celia. "It just made mealtime worse than ever. The doctor told us a stroke sometimes causes muscle weakness or paralysis and loss of sensation in the jaw, gums, and tongue, which can lead to dental problems. In Josh's case his gums had changed."

Although loose dentures can be embarrassing, many physicians recommend that survivors wear their dentures as much as possible during recovery until the jaw and mouth stabilize. After several months Josh's physician and speech therapist determined he was ready to get new dentures.

Routine dental care should also continue after a stroke. You may want to find a dentist who is familiar with treating stroke survivors. Use the guidelines at the beginning of this chapter to help make the best possible choice.

Remember, in addition to ensuring that the survivor receives proper medical and dental care, your role includes incorporating lifestyle changes into the daily life of the survivor and, one would hope, your life as well. Good nutrition, exercise, social activity, and stress reduction are crucial elements for recovery over the long term and can help both of you live healthier, more productive lives. Ways of incorporating these things into your lives are covered in the following chapters.

SIX

Nutrition and Eating Problems

Hard to believe that Abe was practically a gourmet cook before the stroke. Though maybe that was part of what caused it—all those rich sauces and desserts he loved to prepare, and of course eat. Anyway, after the stroke he couldn't even lift a fork, much less prepare a meal. Even after he was physically able to eat again, he just seemed totally uninterested in food. I was so disappointed. When I asked him what the problem was, he just shrugged. I thought maybe my food wasn't appealing enough.

So I decided to take a cooking course to learn how to prepare low-fat meals that could also be tasty. Well, what a difference that made! After my first class I made glazed chicken breast, and Abe actually smiled. He said it was good but that I had cooked it a bit too long.

Pretty soon, after every class Abe would ask me what I had learned. Then he started to modify the menus a bit, suggesting different spices. Within a few weeks he started cooking again! Now we take turns. Our taste buds are still adjusting to these low-fat *dishes, but it's worth it—especially if it can help prevent a stroke from happening again.*

—Ann

Eating can be one of life's greatest pleasures, and losing the ability to feed oneself and enjoy food—even temporarily—can be a very depressing consequence of stroke. One way you as a caregiver can express concern and help the person you're caring for overcome some of these difficulties is by preparing healthful, nutritious meals that look and taste as appetizing as possible— even if at first the survivor's food choices are limited to purees and other easy-to-swallow-and-digest fare.

As in the case of Abe and Ann, you may need to modify your former cooking techniques and allow time to adjust to new tastes and textures. While baked chicken breast won't look or taste like chicken à la king, for example, it can still be a tasty, satisfying dish when prepared with selected herbs and spices. And in learning to cook and plan meals that are low in fat and cholesterol and moderate in calories, you'll have the added satisfaction of knowing that you are contributing to the survivor's recovery and health over the long term (and yours as well!). Following a healthful diet is also an important step in preventing a second stroke (see chapter 9).

In this chapter we'll review how to overcome many of the roadblocks that may stand in the way of the survivor's ability to eat independently, enjoy food, and then reap the benefits of good nutrition. We'll also cover the basics of sound nutrition and offer suggestions for planning meals that are healthful and pleasing.

ROADBLOCKS TO GOOD NUTRITION

After experiencing the physical and emotional trauma of a stroke, the last thing the survivor is likely to have is a hearty appetite. Physical problems that limit his or her ability to use eating utensils or to chew and swallow food, as well as emotional upset, depression, and fears about recovery can interfere with appetite, rob mealtime of its pleasure, and lead to malnutrition. As caregiver, part of your job is to help the survivor regain the ability, motivation, and energy required to maintain good eating habits.

Poor Appetite

Numerous physical and psychological consequences of stroke can cause food and eating to become unappealing to the survivor. As with other conditions related to stroke, identifying the cause of the problem is crucial to finding a solution.

Some of the more common reasons for poor appetite, and strategies for overcoming them, follow:

• Decreased sensation in the mouth, leading to an inability to taste food. Since taste is an integral part of the enjoyment of eating (think about when you have a cold that causes a temporary loss of your ability to taste), it is important to be aware of this factor. Ask the survivor whether he or she can taste food; if not, emphasize the importance of eating regardless of a lack of pleasure in the process.

Have regular discussions with the survivor about the kinds of foods he or she may actually feel like eating and try your best to prepare them, making appropriate substitutions if necessary. For example the survivor might feel like eating ice cream; suggest low-fat frozen yogurt instead.

Try to make the food look attractive—serve puree in a goblet, applesauce in a dessert dish. Atmosphere also counts. Try playing music, lighting candles, or using your best dishes and cloth napkins.

• Fear of choking or embarrassment about chewing and swallowing problems may also cause loss of appetite. Try gentle encouragement: "Take your time, there's no rush, you're doing fine." Also try preparing six daily small meals or snacks instead of three large ones so that the survivor can eat less at one sitting but still get adequate nourishment.

• Depression—or antidepressant medication—may cause a loss of appetite. If the survivor seems depressed, inform your physician or other health professional so that an appropriate treatment plan may be implemented. This may include changing medication, adjusting dosage, and using other strategies to reduce depression such as exercise and social activity (see chapter 7).

• Other medications may also suppress appetite or cause nausea and other gastrointestinal problems that may lead to lack of appetite. Again this situation should be reviewed with your physician and pharmacist so that prescription adjustments may be made.

• Survivors with a short attention span, memory impairment, or confusion may forget about eating even while they are in the middle of a meal, losing interest in their food and walking away from the table. Gently remind these individuals to finish their meal. Minimize distractions in the room while they are eating.

Absorption Problems

As we age, changes occur in the digestive system that may affect how nutrients are absorbed. For example anemia may develop in older adults, who lose the ability to absorb vitamin B_{12} effectively. Medical conditions such as colitis may also affect the body's ability to absorb nutrients. Finally, some of the medications prescribed for stroke-related complications (see chapter 5) may interfere not only with appetite, as described above, but also with the body's ability to absorb nutrients, thus adversely affecting health. Check with your physician or pharmacist to see whether such interactions may affect the survivor's health.

Physical Problems

The problems just mentioned in feeding oneself, chewing, and swallowing may significantly impair the survivor's ability to take in and absorb nutrients. Following the strategies suggested below will help the survivor receive the maximum possible nutritional benefits from each meal.

Feeding Oneself

"I'd say to my mother, 'Mom, finish your dinner,' and she'd just wave her dish away," said Michelle. "I thought she wasn't hungry. But she couldn't tell me that she didn't see the food on the other side of her plate."

Hemianopsia, or the inability to see in half of the visual field (see chapter 4), is one of several problems that can interfere with the survivor's ability to feed himself or herself. Once Michelle realized her mother could not see the food on the right side of her plate, she reminded her to turn her head from side to side. Occasionally Michelle still needs to turn her mother's plate or draw attention to her blind side until looking to either side becomes a habit.

Agnosia, a consequence of stroke that may cause the survivor to use objects inappropriately (see chapter 2), can lead to attempts to eat with fingers or an inappropriate utensil. To assist the survivor in relearning the proper use of utensils, pick up the appropriate utensil, say its name and how it is used, then hand it to the survivor.

Survivors may have to learn to eat with one hand, often the one that is not dominant (i.e., "righties" may need to eat with their left hand). An array of adaptive equipment is available to help the survivor eat more easily during this process. These include the following:

• Built-up handles and universal cuffs, which are devices used by survivors who lack hand strength to help hold utensils. Utensils with built-up handles have large, flexible foam handles wrapped around stainless-steel utensils. A universal cuff can hold different types of utensils and has a band that goes around the survivor's wrist.

• Plate guards that add a metal rim to the outer edge of plates, against which a survivor can scoop food more easily onto a spoon.

• Swivel spoons, used by survivors with wrist problems to help prevent food from spilling out of the spoon.

• Sipper cups, used by survivors with hand-control problems. A sipper cup has a heavy bottom that will right itself and a top to prevent spills.

• Rocker knives, used by survivors who have very limited use of an affected hand. A rocker knife can be used with one hand to cut food.

• Dycem, a two-sided sticky material that helps anchor a plate or tray in place. Nonskid surfaces, such as plastic or vinyl placemats or thin, damp washcloths, may also be used under plates and cups to prevent slipping.

Remember, part of your role in recovery is to help the survivor become as independent as possible. Resist the urge to assist in eating by cutting up food or feeding the person unless he or she is completely disabled.

Chewing

Chewing problems can make eating a difficult, unpleasant experience and may also affect nutrition, since poorly chewed food may not be digested adequately.

If the survivor has trouble chewing, dentures may be needed (or a current pair may fit poorly). Contact your dentist for assistance in diagnosing the problem.

Other reasons for chewing difficulties include poor jaw and tongue movement and loss of sensation in the mouth or tongue. The survivor may be unable to move food to the back of the mouth, a condition called *pocketing*. Again, professional assistance may be needed. In the meantime prepare foods that have a thick, yet soft consistency, such as purees, which are easier to chew than solid foods.

Poor mouth closure caused by weakness in the mouth muscles on the affected side may lead to drooling. In addition to preparing soft food, encourage the survivor to take small bites and to swallow between bites. You can also make things easier by manually helping the survivor to close his or her mouth.

Swallowing

Swallowing problems can be life-threatening (see "Respiratory Complications" in chapter 5). Therefore it is important to be aware of the following symptoms:

- Coughing or choking while eating or drinking
- Wet-sounding voice
- An increase in body temperature one-half to one hour after eating
- Several swallows needed for each bite of food
- Fatigue or shortness of breath
- Congestion in the chest

If you notice any of these symptoms, contact a physician or speech or occupational therapist immediately.

To determine the cause of the problem, a swallowing evaluation may be performed to test the survivor's ability to chew and swallow various types of food and liquid. The problem may be pinpointed by observing how the survivor moves the tongue and lips when chewing and by watching the swallowing process.

If the initial evaluation does not pinpoint the problem, a physician may then conduct a test called a *modified barium swallow,* which is performed in a hospital's

X-ray department. The survivor is asked to swallow a small amount of barium. As he or she swallows, X-ray pictures are taken that show the path that food and liquid take in moving to the stomach. Any factors hindering the process (e.g., lack of muscle contraction in the throat) are identified.

Physical therapists are trained in techniques to stimulate muscle contraction in the throat, jaw, mouth, and tongue. Contact a physical therapist and ask to be shown the exercises used to reeducate the nerves and reflexes that control chewing and swallowing.

General Tips for Eating Independently

"Brenda has many favorite restaurants that we used to go to a lot," says her husband, Carl. *"After her stroke, it was very important for her to regain her dining skills. First she had to adjust to eating with her left hand. She was terribly discouraged at the beginning, when she couldn't even butter a piece of bread. Now we visit some of our old 'haunts' regularly—though we've changed our menu to include mostly low-fat foods."*

In addition to the strategies noted above to deal with specific problems in feeding oneself, chewing, and swallowing, the following tips can be used to help make mealtime more satisfying for the survivor and family members:

• Survivors with impaired neck control or poor posture caused by lack of muscle tone may benefit from supports that hold their head, neck, or back correctly to facilitate feeding and prevent choking. Consult your occupational therapist for suggestions.

• Encourage survivors to use their affected arm when eating finger foods, or holding their napkin to help build strength in that arm.

• Be aware that physical and/or behavioral problems may cause the survivor to spit out food at mealtimes. Contact your physician to determine whether the problem is organic (e.g., reverse swallowing or tongue-thrust problems) or behavioral (e.g., obstinacy, aggression).

• Poor judgment or impaired memory causes some survivors to try to eat or drink too much in one mouthful. Stay alert to such behavior and gently correct it.

• Create a relaxed, festive atmosphere at mealtimes by playing mellow music and placing fresh flowers on the table. It is easier for the survivor to concentrate on eating when the environment is pleasant and free from distractions.

POSTSTROKE NUTRITION: THE BASICS

Once you've helped the survivor to the point where he or she is willing to eat and can do so with some degree of independence, how do you know what to serve? Obviously, relearning the skills necessary for feeding oneself and rekindling appetite should be put to use in the service of a healthful diet rather than a return to junk food or high-fat, high-cholesterol fare.

When the nutritionist told Marie that her husband, Peter, was malnourished, she was confused. "How can

Peter be malnourished?" she asked. "He's overweight. He certainly doesn't look like he's starving."

People may become malnourished even when they are consuming sufficient—or too many—calories.

Like Peter, Sarah has a sweet tooth. "All she wants to eat is candy," says her daughter. "It makes her happy. Shouldn't I let her?"

Calories from foods high in sugar (e.g., candy) or fat (e.g., doughnuts, potato chips) and low in vitamins, minerals, and protein don't provide enough nutrition for good health.

People such as Peter and Sarah would benefit from the dietary guidelines presented in this section. Getting them to follow these guidelines may not be easy, however. Some survivors insist on eating whatever they want. "Why should I deprive myself?" they say.

"I feel like I'm being mean when I tell my husband he can't have ice cream or candy," said Hazel. "But his cholesterol level is way too high. And try as I might, he won't listen to me."

Hazel's problem is not unusual. When the person you are caring for refuses to follow good dietary habits, consult your physician or a registered dietitian. Sometimes encouragement from a medical professional can make a difference.

On the other hand some survivors may understand the vital role diet plays in good health and in stroke prevention and are willing to try foods that held little interest for them in the past. If this is the case with the person you're caring for, take advantage of the survivor's willingness to experiment by preparing these foods in appealing ways. For example serving vegetables with different colors, such as carrots and peas or corn and string beans, can make a meal seem festive; using a variety of spices instead of salt and pepper can add zest to lean meat, poultry, or fish dishes. Contact your local American Heart Association office for booklets with recipes for low-fat meals. And observe the following general guidelines for healthful eating.

Increase Variety

Encourage survivors to eat foods from all food groups, with special emphasis on grains, fruits, and vegetables, as well as low-fat milk and cheese products and low-fat fish, meat, and poultry.

Increase Fiber

Foods in their natural state such as fruits, vegetables, beans, peas, nuts, and whole-grain breads and cereals contain complex carbohydrates and fiber, and generally are more healthful than refined foods, such as most bakery products and candy.

Fiber helps relieve constipation and is associated with reduced risk of heart disease and certain cancers. Fiber also promotes a feeling of fullness, which can help if the survivor is overweight and needs to curb his or her appetite.

Fiber supplements are not recommended unless prescribed by a physician.

Avoid Excess Fat

The intake of saturated fat and cholesterol may contribute to the development of heart disease and a second stroke. To reduce excess fat in the diet:

• Reduce consumption of saturated fats from animal products (beef, pork, lamb, veal, butter, cream, cheese) by trimming fat from meat, removing skin from poultry, and substituting low- or no-fat dairy products for those made with whole milk.

Also avoid saturated vegetable fats—cocoa butter, palm oil, coconut oil—which are often found in bakery items, candies, fried foods, and nondairy milk and cream substitutes.

• Reduce consumption of hydrogenated fats, contained in margarine, some brands of peanut butter, and a wide variety of processed foods, such as crackers and cookies (check ingredients labels when shopping).

• Limit intake of organ meats (liver, sweetbreads), which are very high in fat and cholesterol.

• Broil, boil, bake, or steam foods instead of frying them. Use a spray-on vegetable oil when sautéing.

• Read labels to determine the percentage of fat in foods.

• Try to use products that have fewer than 30 percent of calories from fat.

Avoid Excess Cholesterol

Cholesterol intake should be less than 300 milligrams per day (one egg yolk contains about 213 milligrams of cholesterol—use egg substitutes in baking and don't serve more than three eggs per week). By replacing much of your meat and poultry meals with recipes that emphasize pastas (without creamy sauces), whole grains, vegetables, and fruits, cholesterol (and fat) intake will be dramatically lowered.

Avoid Excess Sugar

Sugar is a source of "empty" calories since it provides no nutrients. To reduce the amount of sugar in the diet:

- Use less of all sugars, including white, brown, and raw sugars, honey, and syrups. None of these forms of pure sugar is significantly better for you than any other.
- Substitute fresh fruit or canned fruit in its own juice or water for sugary foods, such as candy, soft drinks, cake, and cookies.
- Watch for hidden sugars. When reading labels, be aware that sucrose, glucose, dextrose, lactose, fructose, maltose, corn syrup, and corn sweetener are all words that mean sugar. If any of these are among the first ingredients listed on the label, then the product contains a large amount of sugar.

Avoid Excess Sodium

Corinne took the salt shaker off her mother's table and substituted six others: "Pepper, garlic powder, onion powder, dried oregano, dried basil, and an herbal combination—now Mom has taste without the sodium," Corinne says.

Excess salt, either from the salt shaker or in foods naturally high in sodium, increases the risk of hypertension, which is a major factor in heart disease and recurrent stroke.

To limit the amount of salt in the diet, try Connie's suggestion as well as these:

• Add little or no salt to food when cooking.
• Be aware that salt hides under several names. When reading food labels, the word *sodium* means that an item contains salt. Disodium phosphate, monosodium glutamate, sodium chloride, and sodium nitrate are a few of the ingredients that are actually various types of salt compounds.
• Avoid foods with a high salt or sodium content, such as bacon, canned soups and gravies, canned vegetables, potato chips, pretzels, salted nuts, cheese, prepackaged dinners, and many bakery desserts.
• Be aware that many food flavorings are high in salt. Bouillon cubes, chili sauce, garlic salt, onion salt, meat tenderizers, pickles, soy sauce, catsup, and Worcestershire sauce all have a high sodium content (though many of these products are now available in low-salt versions).

Limit Alcohol

Alcoholic beverages, like sugar, are high in calories and low in nutritional value. In addition alcohol—even in moderate quantities—may contribute to physical and mental deterioration in survivors. Limit alcohol consumption to no more than a drink or two daily.

Limit Caffeine

Beverages with a high caffeine content, such as coffee, tea, and cola drinks, also should be consumed in moderation. Caffeine has a stimulating effect on the nervous system that may cause the survivor to become jittery or light-headed. Decaffeinated beverages are rarely caffeine-free, and if consumed in sufficient quantity, even these may cause a caffeine reaction. Instead substitute more healthful liquids, such as water or fruit juice.

Maintain Ideal Weight

Being overweight increases the risk of a number of diseases, including heart disease, hypertension, and diabetes, all of which contribute to the risk of heart attack or recurrent stroke. Excess weight also decreases mobility and interferes with daily activities.

"My husband was stubborn at first," said MaryAnne. "Irv said, 'At my age who cares if I'm fat?'

"I told him I did. Then I got recipes from the dietitian and let Sidney pick out what he wanted me to make. I let Irv know we are in this together. I always eat what he does. And when the kids came over for dinner, they ate the same meals too. I play his favorite music at dinner. And once or twice a week we cheat a little—maybe some ice cream. But best of all, he sees that it works. His cholesterol is way down, he lost weight, and he has more energy. And I feel better too!"

Shopping Tips

• Make a shopping list that includes foods the survivor enjoys.

• Buy a mixture of green leafy vegetables (spinach, mustard or collard greens, kale), cruciferous vegetables (broccoli, brussels sprouts), and yellow vegetables (squash, pumpkin, peppers) to be eaten in salads or steamed as side dishes.

• Buy a variety of fruits (apples, pears, grapes, oranges, bananas) to be eaten raw or cooked for breakfast, snacks, and dessert.

• Don't forget grains, cereals, breads, pasta, rice, potatoes, and other foods high in complex carbohydrates to form the foundation of your meals.

• Try legumes, which are high in protein and low in fat: black, garbanzo, lima, mung, kidney, and pinto beans; black-eyed, yellow, and green peas; lentils and nuts and seeds.

• Stick with low-fat sources of animal protein—chicken, trimmed beef, chicken breast, pork, fish.

• Buy low-fat or nonfat dairy products, including milk, yogurt, and various types of cheeses.

• Avoid prepared foods from the deli counter (potato salad, coleslaw, tuna or chicken salad) since these are generally loaded with oil and mayonnaise.

A registered dietitian or other health professional knowledgeable in nutrition can assist you in planning a weight-loss diet that also provides adequate nutrition for recovery and overall good health. At the same time, you can help the overweight survivor shed excess pounds and maintain ideal body weight by encouraging regular physical activity. The next chapter will tell you how.

SEVEN

Exercise, Socializing, and Other Activities

Mom was always a social butterfly, and the stroke really didn't change that part of her. Even when she was still in a wheelchair, she demanded to go out. I was afraid to let her go, but she's always been independent, even more so since Dad died. So rather than fight with her, I had to figure out how she could get back and forth safely. I couldn't drive her because I had to go to work; it was enough that I had moved into her house to take care of her.

I called the hospital for suggestions, and they advised enrolling her in a stroke club at the local community center. They pick her up and bring her home, plus give her lunch. She loves it! And she's improving so much, soon she won't even need it. She's started going back to the senior center she went to before the stroke, which means I can probably move back to my own home soon. But Mom says she wants to stay in touch with her friends at the stroke center, so we'll arrange that first.

—Don

In this chapter we'll review the benefits of exercise, socializing, and other activities, such as hobbies and traveling, that can help the survivor lead an active life. We'll also cover the skills and equipment needed for survivors who wish to drive again and return to work.

EXERCISE BRINGS MANY BENEFITS

Although the first six months after a stroke is a crucial time for regaining function, improvements in flexibility, coordination, balance, and mobility can continue for months and even years after a stroke.

"When Al's insurance ran out, ending his outpatient therapy after only three months, he was resigned to not even being able to walk down the driveway to get the mail," said his wife, Alice. "But I wouldn't let him accept that. We exercised every day, and six months later he walked to the end of the driveway. After another year he was walking around the yard occasionally. That may not seem like a lot to some people, but for us it is." Alice helps Al by making his home exercise sessions a shared experience. "I put on some music, and we do the exercises together. They're good for me too."

As long as exercise is appropriate to the survivor's medical condition and functional abilities, it can offer numerous physical benefits, such as:

- Increasing and maintaining range of motion
- Increasing flexibility, energy, and stamina

- Improving circulation and decreasing swelling
- Improving coordination and balance

In addition to these overall benefits, exercise also contributes to disease prevention, when other lifestyle modifications are also made:

- In addition to following an appropriate low-fat diet (see chapter 6), quitting smoking, and managing stress, regular exercise can help prevent high blood pressure and heart disease.
- Regular exercise can help the survivor attain and maintain optimal weight and control weight gain. Carrying too much body weight is tiring and is especially detrimental to survivors with heart disease, hypertension, or diabetes (see chapter 6).
- Moderate exercise such as brisk walking for twenty minutes or so several days a week can greatly reduce the risk of a second stroke (see chapter 9).
- Regular exercise brings important emotional benefits. It can help reduce stress and depression while it gives the survivor self-confidence and increased self-esteem.

Because every stroke survivor has different physical needs and limitations, each exercise and activity program should be tailored to the individual. Before a survivor embarks on a new activity or exercise program, a physician and physical and occupational therapists should be consulted to ensure the program will be safe and effective and determine whether the survivor needs to take any special precautions.

STARTING A REGULAR EXERCISE PROGRAM

The success of any exercise program depends upon the survivor's acceptance of his or her current fitness level, the ability to set realistic goals, and a willingness to make slow but steady progress while enjoying the process. To help the survivor achieve exercise success:

• Begin the program slowly and progress gradually, as the individual's condition permits.

• Include a warm-up and cool-down of at least five minutes in each exercise session.

• Include stretching in the program (see page 71 for suggested activities) and, unless the doctor says no, twenty minutes of aerobic exercise three to five times a week.

• Incorporate strengthening exercises two to three times a week unless back pain or other conditions prohibit weight-bearing exercises.

• Set realistic goals that focus on daily activities rather than completing a certain amount of exercise. For example a goal can be to regain enough function to go to the grocery store, play ball with a grandchild, or dance at a son or daughter's wedding. Focusing on a specific return to function can be a powerful motivator for survivors.

General Tips for Regular Exercise

Exercise is an important component of the survivor's recovery program. Ideally the program should include both aerobic exercise and range-of-motion, strengthening, and stretching activities. The following guidelines should be observed when the survivor embarks on a program of regular exercise:

• The program should be started under medical supervision, at least for the first three months following the stroke. This is crucial if the survivor is overweight or has a chronic disease, such as heart disease, hypertension, or diabetes. A thorough medical evaluation should be conducted at regular intervals.

• Ask your physician and pharmacist whether any medications the survivor is taking may alter the body's response to exercise.

• Monitor improvement or backsliding in everyday activities after the exercise program is in place. Report problems to your physician or therapist.

• Keep track of the exercise efforts in a diary. Often improvements are gradual. Survivors may be more motivated and reassured if they can look back and verify that change is indeed taking place.

"Sometimes I feel like I'm not getting any better," says Glenda. "Then I check back three months and see, oh, yes, I only walked for ten minutes then, and now I'm doing twenty. It's nice to see it in black and white."

• Make sure that the survivor takes proper precautions in cold, icy, or snowy weather. Affected limbs get cold easily and need to be properly covered. Wearing multiple layers of clothing helps hold heat next to the body. Survivors who walk with a cane or walker may want to invest in a treadmill at home for the winter months. Some communities have mall-walking programs where the elderly and those with physical limitations can walk during the early-morning hours before stores open.

• Advise the survivor to skip exercise when a fever, flu, or other illness strikes.

• Be aware that inappropriate exercise or overexercising could be detrimental to the cardiovascular system or worsen other chronic diseases.

• Know the warning signs of stroke and cardiac complications (see chapter 9). If these occur, seek immediate medical care.

CHOOSING THE RIGHT TYPE OF EXERCISE

Ideally the survivor should engage in aerobic activities, which stimulate the heart and circulatory system and help burn calories, as well as nonaerobic activities that emphasize flexibility and strength.

Aerobic Activities

Aerobic exercise can help survivors build stamina and endurance. It's important that they select one or more aerobic activities that are pleasant, practical, and fit into their lifestyle.

Walking and Wheeling

Walking is an excellent aerobic activity for many stroke survivors. Sturdy walking shoes are essential. Individuals who need a cane or walker should choose a place that is free of obstacles and has safe areas to sit and rest, such as a park or a mall.

Survivors should not walk alone, especially when

they are first starting their walking program. Some prefer starting out on a treadmill at home or at a health club. These machines are useful in inclement weather or in areas that are not safe for walking. Treadmills with odometers also allow survivors to monitor their own progress.

"My wife, Lydia, and I walk together in a walking club at a neighborhood mall," says Rusty. *"Lydia uses a walker, so it's great to have a safe surface for her, and we can go in any type of weather. We've made so many friends there. Even people in wheelchairs come. It's perfect for them."*

Contact the management personnel in your local malls to see whether they have this type of program. Some hospitals also sponsor walking and wheelchair clubs. A call to a hospital's community-affairs or social worker can put you in touch with such groups.

Jogging

Survivors should not attempt to jog until they have followed a walking regimen for at least twelve weeks. A general guideline to tell if an individual is ready to jog is that his or her walking speed should exceed four miles per hour. Of course the survivor should check with a physician before starting such a program.

Swimming

Swimming is a good aerobic activity for survivors because it is non-weight-bearing, thus the chances of musculoskeletal injury are low. It also requires use of both upper- and lower-body muscles, unlike walking or jogging. Swimming is particularly appropriate for survivors with lower-back problems or balance difficulties.

Many health clubs have pools, as do community centers, YMCA/YWCAs, and some high schools. Check with these facilities to see whether they have special programs for seniors or people with physical limitations. Some community and senior centers offer special water-aerobic or swimming classes for those who need extra assistance.

Cross-country Skiing

Cross-country skiing is a good aerobic activity for some stroke survivors. Like swimming it promotes use of both the upper and lower muscle groups and also improves coordination. Survivors who cannot actually do cross-country skiing may use cross-country-skiing machines, which are an effective way to burn calories and can be used safely indoors in any kind of weather. They are also unlikely to cause musculoskeletal problems.

Cycling

Riding a bicycle requires a good sense of balance and may be beyond the capabilities of many survivors, at least initially. However, some survivors use an adult three-wheeler bicycle, which helps eliminate the problem of maintaining one's balance.

A stationary bike should be used only by individuals who can maintain their balance; otherwise they risk falling forward and injuring themselves. A survivor with relatively good balance and coordination may use a stationary bicycle with a rowing bar, which allows users to work their arms, as well as their legs, in a coordinated motion.

Nonaerobic Activities

Exercises that build strength and increase flexibility and coordination—such as the ones included in home exercise programs from the hospital—are usually nonaerobic. These include basic stretching and flexibility exercises, as well as weight-bearing exercises.

Survivors can add to these basic exercises or substitute other activities, with the permission of their physician or therapist. For example they may use hand weights while walking, or incorporate the use of specific weight machines in their health club activities.

SOCIALIZING

Interacting with people other than caregivers and health care providers is an important part of the survivor's recovery. In the early months after a stroke many survivors are hesitant to have people visit them or to go out. They may feel embarrassed by their physical or perceptual limitations and fearful of rejection. Or they may wish to avoid the pressure of having to interact with others—a chore if the person feels physically weak, unable to carry on a conversation, or unable to concentrate for any length of time.

Nevertheless it is important for them to "reenter the world" as soon as possible. Keeping up with their exercise program is an essential part of the socialization process because it can help give them the confidence they need to be among their friends, family, and strangers again.

Visits from Friends and Family

In the beginning it may be more convenient for survivors to invite people over for conversation, cards, or dinner rather than venturing out into the community. However, it is important to be prepared for possible resistance from friends or family members. Some people are uncomfortable around individuals who have a physical disability. You can ease their discomfort by explaining briefly what they can expect. For example, "Bob speaks very slowly. Just give him a little time," or "Margie can't see things to her right unless she turns in that direction." Giving specifics can allay prospective visitors' "fear of the unknown" and allow them to prepare for the visit.

Pen Pals

It is comforting for survivors to make friendships with people who did not know them before the stroke occurred. These new friends have no preconceived ideas or expectations of the survivor.

For survivors who cannot get out easily, pen pals are an option.

"At sixty-one, my mother just got her first pen pals," says Trudy. *"She writes to one woman in Utah and another in Illinois. They are all stroke survivors. She's thrilled to get mail."*

Survivors can find pen pals in other parts of the United States or in other countries. Some stroke clubs (see below) publish newsletters in which people advertise for pen pals. Individuals who have access to a computer might also try logging on to a computer bulletin board and "conversing" with other people by computer. Contact a local computer club or computer store for information on how to locate and use these systems.

Stroke Clubs

Stroke clubs are a good starting point for survivors who are hesitant about socializing, as well as for their caregivers.

"The camaraderie is wonderful," says Carmela, who started going to stroke-club meetings with her caregiver husband three months after her stroke. "Everyone understands what you're going through, and people accept you as you are. You never have to feel embarrassed about anything. People are patient and kind. I felt like I belonged right from the start. And I've made many new friends."

To find a stroke club in your area, contact the National Stroke Association or call the local chapter of the Easter Seal Society, the American Heart Association, or your hospital social worker or physical or occupational therapist.

Social Groups and Activity Centers

Some community and religious organizations have programs geared to individuals with physical limitations. If you live in a city with a university that has a rehabilitation or gerontology department, contact them to see if they are working on any special projects or activities for stroke survivors.

Many senior-citizen centers, community centers, adult-day-care centers, and stroke-activity centers offer leisure, arts-and-crafts, and exercise programs for the elderly and people with limitations. Some of these facilities also offer lunch and transportation to and from the center, day trips, shopping trips, and other outings. Contact your area Office of Aging or the county department of social services for the location of such services in your community.

Volunteer Organizations

"The day I started volunteering at the children's clinic is the day I began to look forward to getting out of the house," says Marlene, who works two afternoons a week. *"I've made so many friends and met so many caring people. I don't feel sorry for myself like I used to."*

Doing volunteer work can be a very fulfilling activity for the survivor. Marie uses a walker and has limited use of her right hand and arm, but she can do filing and make entries on the computer. Thomas volunteers three mornings a week at a nursing home, where he visits with residents. They and many other stroke survivors find motivation, friendship, and satisfaction from helping others while they help themselves.

Continuing Education

Taking a class is an excellent way for the survivor to learn something new and make new friends. Make sure, however, that the facility is easily accessible (see "Transportation and Accessibility," page 163). Also check with the instructor to see if there are any course requirements that may present problems for the survivor, such as field trips, oral presentations, or use of equipment that requires two hands.

THERAPEUTIC RECREATION

Therapeutic recreation can provide physical or emotional benefits, or both, and often involves socializing with other people. Stroke survivors can participate in dozens of activities. Some decide to take up a new hobby; others need to make adjustments in order to continue with one they enjoyed prior to the stroke.

Horace belonged to a bowling league before his stroke. Now he's in a wheelchair league and uses a special bowling ball with a release handle, for people who have use of only one hand.

Nancy loves to do needlework, but after her stroke she thought she'd never be able to do it again. Her daughter bought her a clamp-on-hoop, which attaches to

Nancy's lapboard. The hoop adjusts to any position and allows Nancy to do needlework with one hand.

Many other devices are available or can be made for survivors who want to pursue hobbies. These include:

- Book holders that permit pages to be turned with one hand.
- Card holders that allow card players to view up to forty cards without having to hold them.
- Clamps and vises that can be attached to tables or lapboards to hold craft items, so that survivors can work on them with one hand. For example Adam uses a vise to hold the wood he uses to carve ducks, and double-sided tape to hold the sandpaper on the workbench.
- Needle threaders that can help those with only one functional hand thread both sewing and yarn needles.
- A special lightweight pusher pool cue stick that allows survivors to play one-handed pool.

Encourage the survivor to investigate a new hobby or take a class in order to learn one. Oil or watercolor painting, Ping-Pong, writing, calligraphy, completing jigsaw puzzles, doing crossword puzzles, gardening, swimming, and gourmet cooking are a few examples of hobbies that can be undertaken without the use of the affected limb. Many computer games can also be played with one hand.

Mind-Stimulating Activities

Michael and Debbie go over all the bills at the end of each month and Michael writes the checks. Even though Debbie cannot write and has trouble reading, she is involved in making decisions about how the household finances are spent.

An active mind is an essential part of rehabilitation and recovery. Involving the survivor in family decision making, even when they cannot actively participate, is an important part of the recovery process.

In addition many hobbies, games, and other activities are therapeutic because they stimulate the mind and help survivors relearn certain skills. Some of these activities are done with other people, so they also increase socialization skills.

Following are some activities to consider:

• Ping-Pong, horseshoes, croquet, and lawn darts, which can improve coordination
• Chess, checkers, and menu planning, which may improve organizational and planning skills
• Games such as cribbage, hearts, and rummy, which can improve concentration and sharpen memory
• Arts and crafts, computer games, and Twenty Questions, which help increase attention span
• Crossword puzzles, Scrabble, bingo, jigsaw puzzles, and paint by number, which help sharpen perceptual skills
• Solitaire and Scrabble, which can promote problem-solving abilities

TRANSPORTATION AND ACCESSIBILITY

Many of the activities described above require the survivor to reenter the community. For reentry to be successful, some planning may need to be done.

For survivors who use wheelchairs, check with your public bus carrier. Some now have hydraulic lifts or ramps that accommodate wheelchairs. Many communities have private handicapped transportation services, and some community and senior-citizen centers have buses that will pick up people who participate in their programs.

Regardless of whether the survivor uses a wheelchair, walker, or cane, call ahead to the destination or check out the location or facility beforehand for the following information:

- Is there accessible parking?
- How far is the parking lot from the building entrance?
- Are there steps that lead into the building? How many? Are there railings? Is there a ramp?
- Is there a revolving door? If so, is there an alternate entryway for the survivor?
- How wide are the doorways? Entranceways need to be at least thirty-two inches wide to accommodate wheelchairs.
- Is there an elevator?
- Are there accessible bathroom facilities? Are there grab bars in the stalls?
- Are the aisles (space between tables, hallways) wide enough for a wheelchair?

TRAVELING

Although traveling to visit friends or relatives or for a vacation can be a welcome—and therapeutic—activity for the survivor, be sure to plan in advance to make the excursion as hassle-free as possible.

Unless you are traveling by car, contact the carrier—cruise ship, airline, bus, train—and let them know you will need special assistance for a wheelchair or an individual using a cane or walker. Most will allow passengers who need assistance to board the aircraft first.

Call ahead to hotels, restaurants, theaters, and attractions to learn whether they have appropriate facilities for a disabled person, as described in the section above. Many hotels now have rooms designed for guests who use wheelchairs, with wide doorways and accessible rest-room facilities.

Following are additional hints to make traveling easier and safer:

• Always clear any travel plans with your physician.
• Use a collapsible walker, which is easier to transport on trains and airplanes.
• Bring a spare cane.
• Request special meals on airlines so that the survivor can follow the healthful guidelines described in chapter 6. Low-fat, low-cholesterol, and vegetarian meals are generally available upon request.
• Make a written request to hotels for special needs: wheelchair access, special meals, room on the lowest floor possible for easy emergency exiting, double beds, grab bars in the bathroom.

• If you check your luggage, always carry on any medications or other vital items in the event your luggage is lost or shipped to another destination. Always carry a list of the survivor's medications and dosing schedules with you.

• Even though you may be planning a restful vacation, be aware that travel is generally stressful, especially for people with physical limitations. Don't plan too many activities. Allow time for rest, and try to keep to the survivor's usual exercise and meal schedules.

DRIVING AGAIN

Being able to drive ensures mobility and independence for the survivor. In many cases it is possible to regain the ability to drive a car safely after a stroke. The key to beginning the process is driver evaluation and training.

Evaluation is the process of examining the extent of the aftereffects of the stroke and determining whether the survivor can be taught or retaught how to drive a vehicle in which special equipment may have to be installed.

A driver's evaluation will usually include:

• Assessment of functional ability
• Reaction-time testing
• Visual testing
• Perceptual testing
• In-car testing

Driver's training may also include:

- In-class instruction
- Classroom driving simulation
- Transfer training
- In-car-on-the-road training
- Wheelchair-loading instruction

It is important to accept that not everyone should get back on the road again. A professional driver evaluation can determine whether driver training is appropriate. Evaluation will also ensure that you do not purchase equipment that is not necessary or unsuitable. Be aware that survivors with perceptual problems (see chapter 2) are less likely to regain safe driving skills.

Nevertheless, with assistance and proper equipment about 80 percent of stroke survivors who attempt to relearn to drive make it back onto the road safely and successfully. To locate a qualified driver-education training program in your area, call your doctor or physical or occupational therapist, or contact your state Office of Vocational Rehabilitation.

Also contact your state motor vehicle office for the forms needed to apply for "handicapped" parking status. Eligibility varies from state to state, but usually requires a form from a physician outlining the extent of the survivor's disability.

Adaptive equipment that can assist in driving again include:

- A spinner knob, which is attached to the steering wheel and permits steering of the car with one hand

- A gas pedal on the left, for the survivor who has limited use of the right leg
- A standard transmission, which is easier to use for survivors who have use of only one lower extremity

RETURNING TO WORK

The desire to return to work—either to a former position or to a new one—is a great motivator for many stroke survivors.

"All Rob talked about was returning to the office," says his wife, Louise. *"But I really didn't know whether he'd be able to do it. He worked as an accountant in a large firm and they gave him a leave of absence after the stroke. But while Rob's mind stayed sharp, he couldn't talk at all for weeks. Finally, four months after the stroke, he was able to make himself understood again.*

"Although it was clear he couldn't return full-time, Rob's boss allowed him to come in once a week for a couple months and handle paperwork—no client contact. Rob was grateful for the chance to return, but he was determined to work with clients again. We redoubled our efforts with the speech exercises and hired a private tutor. Some days I was so exhausted from helping with the exercises that I told Rob to forget it. He'd just tell me to keep quiet and take a rest.

"Now Rob goes in to the office three days a week— and was just given a small client load. It took a lot of hard work, but it was definitely worth it."

Before survivors can return to their previous place of employment or start a new vocation, they need to examine all the physical and mental tasks involved in the job they would like to undertake. This process is called *work-capacity evaluation* and is done professionally in a limited number of places in the United States. Check with your physical and occupational therapists, vocational counselor, or at any university that has a rehabilitation-medicine, biomedical-engineering, physiology, or environmental-health department to see whether they have such a program.

To do your own version of this evaluation, sit down with the survivor and write down all the mental and physical requirements entailed in the job of the person's choice. Items to be considered include how much time he or she must sit or stand, whether any lifting is involved, and how much writing, reading, typing, or mathematical calculations are required.

Next list the survivor's current physical and mental capabilities. A comparison of these two lists will give you and the survivor a fairly realistic idea of how feasible his or her job choice is.

Even if the survivor can return to work, it may be necessary to make changes in the workplace or the work schedule to accommodate the survivor's needs. For example sometimes furniture must be moved or modified to allow for wheelchair access, or individuals may need to sit where they once had to stand. Some people fatigue easily after a stroke and return to work part-time.

Some stroke survivors cannot return to the same job or duties they had before the stroke, but may return to a modified version of their former occupation.

Judith had worked as a field customer service represen-
tative for a telephone company. Her stroke left her par-
tially blind and unable to drive, but she can walk well
with a cane and can communicate well. Because of her
vast experience, she now goes out with customer service
trainees (who drive her to their destination) and teaches
them on the job. She also spends some time in the office
developing training programs.

For some stroke survivors a home office may be an
alternative to returning to work in a business office or
other location. Alternatively the possibility of embark-
ing on a new career may be considered.

William had been a carpenter before his stroke, but
now he uses a walker. Always an active man, he didn't
want to retire at age fifty-eight. Now he operates a busi-
ness from his garage—fixing small appliances—a hobby
he never had enough time to pursue before the stroke.

The process of choosing a new vocation and of coming up with profitable business ideas can be interesting
and fun. Help the survivor start with activities you
know he or she enjoys, and move forward from there. A
new vocation may end up being more rewarding than
the old one!

HOMEMAKING

"I always joked with my husband that watching him
try to do housework was motivation enough for me to

regain as much of my faculties as possible," says Carolyn.

Returning to homemaking is an important step for many stroke survivors because it is a sign of independence. As they begin doing homemaking activities again, they may discover that their physical strength and stamina are not what they used to be. Try to arrange chores so that they can be done safely, with a minimal amount of effort.

General Tips for Working in the Home

To promote as much independence as possible on the part of the survivor, encourage him or her to:

• Plan ahead. Have everything needed for a specific task in one place to eliminate extra movement.
• When possible, slide items rather than lifting them.
• Break down large tasks into smaller ones. It isn't necessary to do all four loads of laundry in the same day.
• Avoid heavy lifting.
• If possible, sit when performing tasks.
• Work at a comfortable height. Unnecessary leaning or bending can cause fatigue or loss of balance.
• Work at a moderate pace and rest frequently.
• Alternate between light tasks (washing dishes, folding laundry) and heavy chores (making beds, vacuuming, mopping the floor).
• Rest frequently.

Adaptations can be made around the house to make cleaning easy and safe. Suggest that the survivor

- Use a utility cart to transport items around the house
- Use a vacuum cleaner that rolls easily and has extendable attachments
- Use long-handled tongs or reachers to pick up items from the floor
- Attach long handles to sponges or dust mops to clean hard-to-reach places
- Use buckets on rollers
- Sit while sorting and folding laundry
- Sit while ironing

Meal preparation will go more smoothly and safely if the following guidelines are heeded:

- Place frequently used items on shelves and in drawers that are easily accessible.
- Hang cooking utensils on a wall or pegboard at chest or head level for ambulatory survivors, lower for survivors who use wheelchairs.
- Store dishes in a vertical position for easier access.
- Use a cutting board with nails driven into it so that fruits and vegetables stay secure during peeling and cutting.
- Turn handles of pots and pans away from the front of the stove to avoid accidents.
- Simplify the menu: Make one-dish meals, use healthful prepared or frozen foods when possible (allowing of course for dietary needs).
- Use electrical appliances such as can openers and

food processors rather than those that require hand labor.

• Use kitchen appliances and tools designed for people with limited hand function. See the appendix for sources of these items.

Body Mechanics That Save Energy

Help survivors who want to return to useful activity to:

• Sit and stand correctly, keeping the body aligned.

• Work at a comfortable height to minimize stooping, bending, or reaching.

• Arrange work so that arms can be held close to the body.

• Lift objects by standing with knees bent and maintaining a feeling that their weight is centered in the lower body. Most of the work should be done by the quadriceps, the large muscles in the thighs, not the arms or the lower back.

• Use the muscles and joints best suited for the job. For light work this means not using more parts of the body than necessary. For heavy work this means using the largest and strongest muscles, such as the thighs and buttocks.

Leading an active life and making beneficial use of time can be powerful motivators for you and the survivor alike. By helping the survivor make the most of his or her physical and mental capabilities and encouraging reentry into the community, you will undoubtedly contribute to the survivor's recovery.

You're also more likely to enjoy being with the survivor when he or she is alert, motivated, and taking an active role in the recovery process. This can be particularly important during the times when you take a much-needed break from caregiving. The next chapter will help you learn how to make the most of your leisure time.

EIGHT

Taking a Break From Caregiving

"Sometimes I wish someone would call me on the phone and say, 'Sally, I'll come over and stay with Bill for the afternoon. You go to a movie.' That would be wonderful!"

When friends stop over, they stay a few hours, then tell Ethel, "Bob doesn't seem to be bad at all."

"But they aren't with him twenty-four hours a day, seven days a week," Ethel says. "Just being there, always alert to his needs, is tiring and stressful. He gets depressed and cries. I worry that he'll fall or have another stroke. They don't see any of that."

"Now that Rose can't do much of the housework, I do the work of two people," says Stu. "I had to take a crash course in cleaning, cooking, laundry, and everything else. Our lives have changed entirely. But we try to keep a sense of humor about everything. Maybe that's what keeps us going."

"When you need people to keep you from getting depressed, to relieve you once in a while, and just be

there for you—that's when you find out who your
real friends are," Karen says. "You can't be afraid to
admit you need help. You have to ask, and know it's
really the best thing you can do for yourself and for
the survivor."

Like you, these people are caregivers—a spouse, son, daughter, relative, or friend who has been entrusted with the care of a stroke survivor. Every day you face the challenges, frustrations, and rewards that such care entails. In the process you may forget that you need to take care of yourself too.

This chapter is just for you. In it we cover the caregiver's "survival" strategy, which consists of three basic elements: acceptance, communication, and action. By implementing this strategy you can learn to deal with your feelings—negative as well as positive—and obtain relief from the emotional and physical stresses of caregiving.

ACCEPTING YOUR ROLE

An important concept to embrace as a caregiver is acceptance: you need to accept the fact that you have undertaken this role, which entails many responsibilities. Acceptance means you acknowledge the reality of your situation and are doing something about it. It does not mean you have to like it, nor does it mean that you accept it every moment of every day.

As we saw in chapter 1, in many cases caregivers do not volunteer for the role: your spouse, parent, or another relative or friend has a stroke, and the job of caregiver is suddenly thrust upon you. Accepting your role makes it easier to move forward because you can stop spending energy on fighting the situation.

Acceptance also means accepting your feelings, which may include feelings you believe you "shouldn't" have, such as anger, feeling trapped, depression, fear, insecurity, and loneliness. Yet these feelings are perfectly normal. If you accept that these "negative" feelings go hand in hand with caregiving, you won't feel guilty for experiencing them, and they won't destroy the warm, caring, and giving feelings you also have.

"At first I kept saying, 'Why me?' " says Pauline. " 'Why did my husband do this to me?' Of course I knew it wasn't his fault, but I was so angry and hurt. I felt like someone had robbed me of my life."

Acceptance is an ongoing process. One day you'll feel like you can cope and the next you'll be saying, "I can't take it." This, too, is natural.

"Every morning I say a little prayer," says Pauline. "First I'm thankful that Charles and I can be together. Then I ask for the strength and patience to get through another day."

COMMUNICATING YOUR NEEDS AND EMOTIONS

"You have to let the survivor and others around you know that you are a person with needs too," says Lester. "That means you need time for yourself—to be

alone or to socialize with friends. If you don't say any-thing, or feel guilty about taking that time, you'll only hurt yourself and the survivor in the long run."

The second survival element involves keeping lines of communication open and clear between yourself and the survivor. Let him or her know that you intend to take care of yourself, too, as well as the steps you will take to ensure that your needs get met. This may mean having a friend or relative come in while you go out for a few hours, or setting aside a half hour or so daily to take a walk or meditate. Or it may mean that you occasionally take the survivor to an activity center or residential day-care center while you go shopping or spend time with friends.

Communication also involves expressing your needs to those who are close to you. Share your feelings and concerns; ask for help when you need it and accept help from those who offer it. Seek out people who are willing to learn what the caregiver role is about and occasionally assist in the process. Loyal, understanding friends and family can be important resources.

Following are some techniques for coping with feelings related to caregiving.

Anger

Anger is probably the most common emotion experienced by caregivers. Accept that you will feel angry at various times and to varying degrees. You may end up directing your anger at the survivor, yourself, relatives or friends who may not be supportive, or other members of the stroke-recovery team (see chapter 1).

"Sometimes I get so angry at Charles, I snap at him," says Pauline. *"Then I feel guilty about making him feel bad. I'm not really angry at him; I'm angry at the stroke and what it's done to our lives. But I feel like I need to lash out at someone, and no one else is here."*

Misdirected anger—lashing out at the stroke survivor or other people, or chastising yourself—can place strains on your emotional and physical health and on your relationships. On the other hand repressed anger can lead to depression and fatigue and may exacerbate physical ailments such as stomach disorders and head-ache. To direct your anger in a healthier way, try the following:

• Discuss your feelings with someone who is not directly involved with your situation—a minister, thera-pist, social worker, or close friend.

• Remove yourself from the situation, even if only briefly. "Sometimes I just want to scream," say many caregivers. Some of them do—they go into their rooms and scream into a pillow. Or try what Peggy does: She drives down a country road with the radio blaring while she screams as loudly as she can. The key is to separate yourself from the survivor and go to a safe place—the garden, your room, the bathroom, the base-ment—and take time for yourself. Punch a pillow, listen to classical music, play the piano, relax in a hot bath, read poetry, take deep breaths.

• Share your anger occasionally in a constructive way with the survivor. He or she needs to know that you are human too. If you are angry at someone other than the survivor—a relative who promised to come over and then canceled, or service people who won't return your phone calls—say what you're feeling and why, otherwise the survivor may think he or she is the cause of your anger.

• Avoid self-destructive behaviors. Turning to drugs, alcohol, cigarettes, or food in order to "drown" your feelings will only make you feel worse in the long run.

• Incorporate regular exercise into your life, especially some form of vigorous activity that can help you release pent-up anger safely (check with your physician before starting a new exercise program). Ethel bought an aerobic tape that she pops into the VCR whenever she feels the need to let go. Some caregivers take brisk walks or join an exercise class.

Guilt

Am I doing enough? Am I a selfish person if I want to go out occasionally? What if I leave my mother with a friend and something happens while I'm out? What will people think if I don't stay with my husband twenty-four hours a day?

Guilt is an emotion that can easily get out of hand. Many caregivers believe they must be superhuman.

"I thought I always had to be cheerful," says Irene. "I didn't want Will to see that I was depressed or tired. I thought I wasn't being supportive enough if I let him see the downside of my feelings."

In fact caregivers who act this way are hurting the survivor and themselves more than helping. When Irene shared her feelings in her caregiver support group, the other members helped set her straight. "They showed

me that I shouldn't feel guilty about how I felt," Irene
says. "I'm doing the best I can, and I deserve some rest
and recreation. The group told me, no one is perfect, so
stop applying for the job!"

The next time you feel guilty, consider the following:

• Did you yell at the stroke survivor or a friend or
relative for no justifiable reason? Okay, accept that
you're human. Apologize and try implementing some of
the strategies above.
• Did someone say something to you to make you
feel like you're not doing enough or that your job is
"easy"? Recognize that most people who make insensi-
tive remarks usually don't understand how much energy and time is required of a caregiver.
• Did you go out with friends and feel guilty when
you got home? If you left the survivor in capable hands,
you have no reason to feel guilty. You deserve time to
reenergize and unwind. You will be much more effective and helpful to the stroke survivor if you take care
of yourself.

Feeling Trapped or Helpless

Rhoda, age sixty-three, was working as a legal secre-
tary in a large law firm until her husband, David, had a
stroke. She took early retirement in order to stay home
to care for him. For the first few months she was filled
with a deep sense of hopelessness and despair.

"I was suffocating," Rhoda says. "I was afraid to go
out because I thought he might have another stroke. I

pictured the two of us sitting in the house and fading away. I figured we'd never travel again, never do all the things we had planned for retirement. We were still young enough to enjoy life, yet we were trapped."

Rhoda's sense of hopelessness made her believe there was no way out. She became depressed. Fortunately her daughter visited from out of state and convinced her to see a counselor. She also took Rhoda to a support group. Soon Rhoda began to see her situation in a different light, even though David's condition had not changed. Now she has a home companion come in three mornings a week while she goes to work part-time —and she and David are planning to take a cruise.

Fear and Frustration

Fear of the unknown—if another stroke will occur, if the survivor will fall, if your son or daughter may also have a stroke at a young age—is common among caregivers. Again, caregiver support groups are an excellent place to air these fears and get reassurance.

Florence remembers when she went to her first caregiver support group. "The first question I wanted someone to answer was 'What do I do if he has another stroke?' and the chorus of responses was 'You'll get through it.' They had all experienced the same fear. I wasn't alone. It was comforting to know that these people would be there for me if it happened."

Frustration can come from various circumstances. The survivor may refuse to accept help or care from anyone other than the caregiver. You may also experience frustration if the survivor seems to be giving up, or refuses to participate in therapy. Seek professional assistance if these situations occur, since they can be destructive to you and to the survivor.

Depression

"For the first few months I was so overwhelmed with the new responsibilities, I didn't have much time to think about myself," says Murray. "When we got into an hour-by-hour, day-to-day routine, I realized I was incredibly sad and lonely. Jane needed a lot of care, and I was willing to give it. But I was depressed all the time, and that wasn't helping either of us. She wasn't motivated to do her exercises, and neither was I. I knew this wasn't good."

Murray knew he needed help with his depression. He tried some of the suggestions in the sections above, which are effective for many caregivers. But when he realized that was not enough, he sought other solutions.

A retired store manager, Murray had always had an interest in photography. He signed up for photography classes two mornings a week and brought in a home health care worker for those times. When he saw that Jane was comfortable with the arrangement—"In fact," he says, "she was glad to have someone else to talk to besides me!"—they decided she would go to a day-care center two days a week so that she could socialize with others. They both felt better, and Jane started making progress again.

TAKING ACTION

Action includes whatever steps you take to cope with the stress associated with your caregiver's duties, such as those suggested above. Plus it's important to join a caregiver support group. "It's the best thing I ever did," says Harriet. "The amount of caring and understanding I get from the other group members is unbelievable. Every caregiver should go to one of these groups." (See chapter 10 for resources.)

Following are some additional suggestions for ways of coping with the stress of caregiving:

• Solicit and accept offers of help from family and friends. Don't feel guilty about "burdening" them.

• Don't let people criticize your caregiving activities. "What do you do all day?" is a question some caregivers hear from relatives or friends. "Unless they've done it themselves," says Stu, "most people don't realize that caregiving means that you—or someone else—have to be there for the stroke survivor twenty-four hours a day. You have to plan and schedule everything, because you can't afford to forget anything. If Tuesdays and Fridays are the only days you can get out to the store and you forget to buy bread on Tuesday, you're out of bread and out of luck!"

"All the little things you do add up," adds Peggy. "When people ask me what I do all day, I pull out my lists and schedules and show them: medication times, doctors' appointments, exercise times, meals, cleaning, errands. That keeps them quiet."

• Find an outlet in the community just for you: attend a class, join a social or church group.

• Although there will be times when you cannot get out of the house, don't let yourself become isolated. Use the telephone to stay in touch with relatives and friends. Invite people over—friends, neighbors, relatives, your minister. Get a pet. Write letters. Listen to call-in talk-radio shows.

• Maintain your personal appearance. If you look good, you'll feel better.

• Keep a diary or journal and write down how you feel each day. Seeing it in black and white can give you a better perspective.

• If you have a computer and modem, join an on-line support network.

• Seek spiritual guidance if this helps you.

PRIVATE AND COMMUNITY CAREGIVING SERVICES

There are several alternatives for long-term, ongoing relief for caregivers. Some involve people coming to your home; others require that you take the survivor to a facility on a regular basis. Following are some of the types of options to consider. (See chapter 10 for specific resources.)

Home Visits

Friendly Visitors
These are volunteers who visit people in their homes for several hours a week. Their primary purpose is to provide companionship and conversation and help sur-

vivors with reading or letter writing. They do not clean or perform any personal or medical tasks, and the service is usually free.

Senior Companions

"A senior companion has been a lifesaver for me," says Fred. "My wife can get around the house, but I need someone there during the day while I'm working in case she falls. The companion makes lunch for Pat, and they play cards, watch television, write letters. She's great company for Pat."

Senior companions are trained to provide minimal services, such as prepare meals and monitor the survivor's safety. They do not help with bathing or personal hygiene or do any housecleaning or heavy lifting. Costs depend on the area.

Licensed Home Health Care Personnel

Home health aides, registered nurses, and homemakers are available through health care agencies (see chapter 1, page 15). Use an agency licensed by your state's department of health. Depending on your needs, the agency can send you an individual who will do housecleaning, cooking, shopping, personal-care chores such as bathing and toileting, and dispense medications. Costs vary, and some insurance companies will pay for such services.

Be aware that nursing care will be reimbursed by Medicare for a limited time only, if such care is ordered by a physician. In most cases the services of the nurse must be supplied through a home health agency that is in accord with Medicare guidelines.

Physical, Occupational, and Speech Therapists

Reimbursement under Medicare and Medicaid may be available when these services are provided in the home. Therapists are available through certified home-care agencies or from private practices. In general the survivor must be making progress toward defined goals that the therapists and survivor have discussed and agreed upon. Reimbursement by third parties will usually not be provided if the individual has reached a functional plateau, and the sessions merely help to maintain that level. For more on the roles of these therapists, see chapter 1.

Community-Based Services

Community-based services can often provide a much-needed break by offering the caregiver an opportunity to take the survivor to a facility and leave him or her there for several hours or a full day.

Adult Day Care

This is a relatively new concept in rehabilitation that is intended to supplement the care given by the family at home and provide an alternative to nursing-home care. For Helen an adult-day-care center provided the ideal solution. She desperately wanted to return to work part-time but felt guilty about leaving her husband, John, home alone, and he refused to have "a stranger" in the house. John was able to get around quite well with a walker, but he said he didn't like to go out. When Helen told him the adult-care center was having a John Wayne film festival, she knew he couldn't resist seeing his movie idol. Once he met the other people at the center, he agreed to go back. Now he spends five mornings a week there while Helen goes off to work.

Be aware that the services in these centers can vary greatly. They may offer nursing and counseling services as well as therapeutic and recreational activities from one to five days a week, usually from three to six hours a day. Transportation and hot meals may also be provided.

Senior Center

Senior center is a term loosely used to cover any of a number of community centers, often associated with churches or civic groups, that provide recreational activities for older adults. In many cases these organizations do not provide nursing or other health or medical care, though staff may be trained in working with seniors who have a wide range of disabilities. Before enrolling the survivor in a senior center, meet with the staff to see whether they are equipped to handle any special needs the survivor may have and whether the survivor's level of recovery would permit him or her to participate effectively in the activities offered.

Respite Care

The word *respite* comes from the Latin *respirare,* "to breathe." It can work in one of two ways: You can take the survivor to a hospital or nursing home that has such a program, or else a member of the program comes to your home and stays with the survivor while you're out.

"Boy, did we need a breather!" says Lloyd. "Caring for my mother was a tremendous strain on both me and my

wife, Claudia. The respite program at our hospital took care of my mother for a week while Claudia and I took a vacation. It was reassuring to know that she was getting all the attention and care she needed. We'll use them again when we need another break."

Respite costs generally are not covered by insurance plans. In some communities church and civic groups offer respite care. These programs are staffed by volunteers for a nominal fee.

Call your local area Office of Aging for information on supportive services in your community. Look in the phone book for the number of this office or your state office on aging. Also consult the organizations listed in the Resource Guide for additional help.

NINE

Preventing a Second Stroke

After Marcia's stroke, the social worker at the hospital warned me that one of the biggest fears people have is that it might happen again. Marcia was afraid she'd get another one, and believe me, I was scared to death it might happen to me. I read everything I could about stroke prevention, and followed the advice of our physician. So far it seems to have worked. Alice is healthy now, and I'm still feeling fine. But I know all the changes we've made, such as quitting smoking and exercising several times a week, are part of a new lifestyle. We can't ever go back to our old bad habits.

—*Jerome*

A major concern of anyone who has suffered a stroke —as well as for the person caring for the survivor—is that it may happen again. This is a very real concern, since studies show that approximately 25 percent of stroke survivors suffer a second stroke. Therefore in this chapter we will cover the signs and symptoms that may occur prior to a second stroke, explain how a stroke happens, and review the steps you can take to help the survivor avoid a second stroke.

STROKE WARNING SIGNS

There are specific physical and mental changes associated with an impending stroke. These warning signs should prompt you to call 911 or the emergency department of your local hospital immediately so that appropriate measures may be taken. The survivor should also review these symptoms and be told to call the hospital immediately if he or she experiences them; the signs that preceded the first stroke might have been somewhat different (since symptoms may occur alone or in combination).

By recognizing the warning signs and taking immediate action, a second stroke may be averted or, if it does occur, its severity may be reduced. They are as follows:

• Numbness, weakness, or paralysis of the face, arm, or leg, occurring on one or both sides of the body
• Sudden blurred or decreased vision in one or both eyes
• Difficulty speaking or understanding simple statements
• Sudden severe headache
• Difficulty swallowing
• Sudden difficulty with memory, judgment, or orientation
• Dizziness, loss of balance, or an unexplained fall when combined with another warning sign

Some strokes are preceded by warning signs called *transient ischemic attacks TIAs),* or ministrokes. TIA symptoms are similar to the symptoms of a full-blown stroke, except that they generally disappear within twenty-four hours, since TIAs are caused by a temporary, not permanent, interruption of blood flow within an artery leading to the brain.

Again, recent research confirms that a stroke or TIA should be treated as a medical emergency; do not wait a day or so to see whether symptoms disappear. By getting the stroke survivor to the hospital after a TIA, a stroke recurrence may be prevented.

Related changes in the survivor's condition that should also be reported to a physician because they may precede a TIA or stroke include: elevated blood pressure, nosebleeds, unexplained headaches, visual disturbances, irregular pulse, mood changes, temporary weakness in an arm or leg not affected by the stroke, temporary memory loss, temporary loss of consciousness.

WHAT HAPPENS DURING A STROKE

What happens in the body to cause such symptoms? A stroke is defined as a sudden, often severe impairment of the body caused by a disruption in the flow of blood to the brain. When blood can't get through to areas of the brain, the supply of oxygen and nutrients to the brain cells in these areas is cut off. The affected brain cells become damaged or die.

Disruption of blood flow can be caused by blockage

or constriction of a cerebral (brain) or carotid (neck) artery, or by the bursting of a section of a cerebral artery, causing bleeding into the brain.

Types of Stroke

There are two main types of stroke: ischemic and hemorrhagic. *Ischemic strokes*—which include thrombotic and embolic strokes—occur when there is a sudden cutoff in the flow of blood to an artery in the brain, causing brain cells to become damaged or die due to lack of oxygen.

A *thrombotic stroke,* also known as *cerebral thrombosis,* is caused by a clot that forms in an artery in the brain. This is usually due to atherosclerosis—the buildup of fatty deposits in the arteries. The clot—formed when blood cells stick to these deposits—blocks the artery, stopping the flow of blood. This is the most common type of stroke, and accounts for about 60 percent of all strokes.

An *embolic stroke* is caused by a clot that forms in an artery in another part of the body, such as the heart. A piece of the clot, called an *embolus,* breaks loose and travels through the bloodstream to the brain, where it gets stuck in a small blood vessel, plugging up the vessel and cutting off the blood supply. This sudden blockage, called an *embolism,* accounts for approximately 20 percent of strokes.

Hemorrhagic strokes—which include *intracerebral hemorrhage* and *subarachnoid hemorrhage,* named for the area of the brain in which they occur—is caused by blood leaking into brain tissue from a ruptured blood vessel. Blood vessels may rupture as a result of high blood pressure, a weak spot in the artery wall *(aneurysm)*, or malformations of the vessels.

Hemorrhagic strokes are less common than ischemic strokes. Intracerebral hemorrhage accounts for approximately 12 percent of strokes, and subarachnoid hemorrhage is responsible for approximately 8 percent of strokes.

REDUCING STROKE RISK FACTORS

In addition to watching for stroke warning signs, it is important to minimize the chance that a second stroke will occur by helping the survivor to reduce stroke risk factors.

Some risk factors cannot be changed. These include age, gender, race (blacks have a higher incidence of high blood pressure and stroke than Caucasians), family and individual history of stroke or TIA, and diabetes.

However, many risk factors can be changed, including treatable medical disorders and lifestyle. Most of these steps are covered in earlier chapters, since part of the treatment of stroke involves curbing risk factors. We'll review these steps here, with an emphasis on their importance for preventing a second stroke.

Remember, the steps outlined in this section should be followed not only by the stroke survivor but by you and other family members as well. By helping the survivor reduce the risk of having another stroke, you also help reduce your own stroke risk.

Hypertension

Keep high blood pressure under control by following a low-fat, low-sodium diet, limiting alcohol consumption, and taking medication as prescribed. Medication to control hypertension is effective only if taken on a regular basis, even on days when the survivor is feeling well. High blood pressure may contribute to as many as 90 percent of strokes.

Weight and Exercise

A desirable weight is maintained by following an appropriate diet and exercising regularly. Being overweight strains the heart and blood vessels and is associated with high blood pressure. Obesity also predisposes to heart disease and diabetes, both of which—like high blood pressure—increase the risk for stroke.

Regular exercise helps keep weight down, reduces the risk of heart disease (and thus stroke), and can reduce stress.

Smoking

Stop smoking. In addition to harming the lungs, cigarette smoking also injures blood vessel walls, speeds up hardening of the arteries, and elevates blood pressure. Studies suggest smokers have a three-times-greater risk of stroke than nonsmokers. The stroke risk for smokers who also have high blood pressure can be as much as twenty times greater than for nonsmokers. Stroke risk declines for those who stop smoking, regardless of how much, and for how long, they have smoked in the past (see chapter 10 for organizations that offer stop-smoking programs).

Atrial Fibrillation

People with atrial fibrillation, a heart condition in which the heart beats in an irregular fashion, have a significantly higher risk of stroke or a second stroke. Recent studies suggest that the drug warfarin reduces stroke rate in these individuals. Discuss this option with your physician.

Aspirin

Aspirin is one of several antiplatelet agents that have been investigated to see whether their use can help prevent thrombus formation (see pages 111 and 192) and reduce stroke risk. Although results are not definitive, several recent studies have demonstrated that low doses of aspirin can be effective in preventing stroke after a TIA. Discuss this option with your physician.

Ticlopidine

Ticlopidine is another antiplatelet agent. It has been found to be more effective than aspirin for the reduction of thrombotic stroke in people who have experienced stroke symptoms and to reduce the risk of recurrent stroke. Ticlopidine is a prescription drug and should be discussed with your physician.

Oral Contraceptives

Oral contraceptives can increase the risk of blood clots and emboli—potential causes of stroke—especially in women over age thirty. The risk is higher for women who also smoke. Your physician can suggest alternative birth control methods for women in either of these categories.

Stress

Although a certain amount of stress is inevitable, studies suggest that stress contributes to high blood pressure and, by extension, the risk of stroke. By managing stress with exercise, relaxation techniques, and counseling if needed, stroke risk may be reduced.

A FINAL WORD ABOUT STROKE RECOVERY

After a stroke there is rarely any "going back." But there is always an untraveled path in front of the person who has survived a stroke and the people who are caring for the survivor. By now you are probably well along this road, which, while long and difficult, is one that has been successfully traveled by millions of survivors and caregivers. Many, many stroke survivors have made full or nearly full recoveries—and the person you care for can be among them.

We hope that this book will help make the fullest possible recovery a reality for you and for the survivor.

TEN

Stroke Resource Guide

NATIONAL STROKE ASSOCIATION

National Stroke Association (NSA) is the primary resource organization for stroke-survivor and caregiver support and for patient, public, and professional education. Founded in 1984, NSA is a national voluntary health care organization and the world's largest provider of stroke-related materials. Its services include the following:

Stroke Survivor and Caregiver Support

• NSA connects stroke survivors and caregivers with stroke support groups in communities across the nation.

• *Be Stroke Smart,* NSA's quarterly newsletter, reports on progress and issues in stroke prevention, research, treatment, rehabilitation, and survivor and caregiver support.

• NSA's Stroke Information and Resource Center is a national clearinghouse of information on stroke statistics, medical referral sources, support groups for survivors and caregivers, rehabilitation facilities, and manufacturers and distributors of adaptive resources and equipment.

Patient and Public Education

• NSA provides stroke data, information, and sources to national media.

• NSA sponsors public education programs using print and audiovisual materials to inform the public about stroke prevention through management of stroke risk factors, recognition of stroke warning signs, and getting emergency medical treatment when warning signs occur.

• NSA's Stroke Prevention Screening Program provides hospitals and other organizations with information and tools to conduct public screenings to identify and counsel those at risk for stroke.

Professional Education

• NSA publishes *Journal of Stroke and Cerebrovascular Diseases,* a quarterly medical journal, and *Stroke: Clinical Updates,* a bimonthly medical publication.

• NSA sponsors symposia and other programs on stroke for the medical profession.

• NSA provides physicians and other health care professionals with patient education materials on stroke prevention, treatment, and rehabilitation.

NSA National Office

National Stroke Association
8480 East Orchard Road, Suite 1000
Englewood, CO 80111-5015
Phone: 1-800-STROKES (1-800-787-6537) or (303) 771-1700
Fax: (303) 771-1886
TDD: (303) 771-1887

NSA Chapters
Harmarville Rehabilitation Chapter of the National Stroke
Association
P. O. Box 11460
Guys Run Road
Pittsburgh, PA 15238-0460

Contact: Ann Boyle, R.N., Chapter Coordinator, (412) 826-
2737

Minnesota Chapter of the National Stroke Association
910 East 26th Street, Suite 210
Minneapolis, MN 55404

Contact: Liz Greeman, Chapter Exec. Director, (612) 879-
0015

Rocky Mtn. Stroke Chapter of the National Stroke
Association
4500 East Iliff Avenue
Denver, CO 80222

Contact: Esther Fretz, (303) 782-5831

South Florida Chapter of the National Stroke Association
North Broward Medical Center
201 East Sample Road
Pompano Beach, FL 33064

Contact: Barbara Brown, Chapter Exec. Director, (305) 786-
7333

GENERAL RESOURCES

ABLEDATA and NARIC
8455 Colesville Road, Suite 935
Silver Spring, MD 10910-3319
(301) 588-9284 (V/TT)
(800) 227-0216 (V/TT)
(301) 589-3563 BBS

An electronically maintained database of information on assistive technology: product descriptions, manufacturer addresses and phone numbers, and pricing. Anyone may access the information by calling, writing to, or visiting the company's office; purchasing the database on CD-ROM or diskettes; or using the ABLE INFORM Bulletin Board System (BBS).

Alzheimer's Association
919 North Michigan, Suite 1000
Chicago, IL 60611-1676
(312) 335-5776
(312) 335-8882—TDD

A national nonprofit organization dedicated to research for the prevention, cure, and treatment of Alzheimer's disease and related disorders and to providing support and assistance to afflicted patients and their families. The association works through a network of 221 chapters, 1,600 support groups, and more than 35,000 volunteers nationwide.

American Association of Homes for the Aging
901 East Street, N.W., Suite 500
Washington, DC 20004
(202) 783-2242

Represents not-for-profit organizations dedicated to providing quality health care, housing, and services to the nation's elderly through interaction with Congress and federal agencies. Enhances the professionalism of practitioners and facilities, holds conferences, and provides publications. Free catalog.

American Association of Retired Persons (AARP)
601 East Street, N.W.
Washington, DC 20049
(202) 434-AARP

Health care information and publications on subjects such as caregiving, insurance, safety, long-term care, and so on. Some available on audiotapes, videotapes, and in Spanish. Write for free catalog. No orders via phone.

American Diabetes Association
1660 Duke Street
Alexandria, VA 22314
(703) 549-1500

The nation's leading voluntary health organization supporting diabetes research and education. Founded in 1940 as a medical society, the association has an affiliate office in every state and activities in more than eight hundred communities nationwide.

American Foundation for the Blind
3342 Melrose Avenue, N.W.
Roanoke, VA 24017
(800) 829-0500

Products for people who are blind or visually impaired. Free catalog.

American Health Care Association
1201 L Street, N.W.
Washington, D.C. 20005
(202) 842-4444

National trade association representing U.S. long-term-care facilities.

American Heart Association/Stroke Connection
7272 Greenville Avenue
Dallas, TX 75231
(800) 553-6321

Provides services to stroke survivors and caregivers, such as information and referral, materials, newsletters, and stroke-club support. For information call the above number or your local American Heart Association.

American Occupational Therapy Association
1383 Piccard Drive
P. O. Box 1725
Rockville, MD 20849-1725
(301) 948-9626
(800) 377-8555—TDD

American Physical Therapy Association (APTA)
1111 North Fairfax Street
Alexandria, VA 22309
(703) 684-2782

A national professional organization representing more than fifty-six thousand physical therapists, physical-therapist assistants, and physical-therapy students throughout the United States. Its goals are to increase the understanding of the therapist's role in the health care system and to foster improvements in physical-therapy education, practice, and research.

American Printing House for the Blind, Inc.
P. O. Box 6085
Louisville, KY 40206-0085
(502) 895-2405

Produces products for the visually impaired—Braille, large print, talking books and magazines, and educational and daily-living aids. Free catalog and newsletter.

American Public Health Association
1015 15th Street, N.W.
Washington, DC 20005
(202) 789-5600

American Society on Aging
833 Market Street, Suite 512
San Francisco, CA 94103
(415) 882-2910

American Speech-Language-Hearing Association
10801 Rockville Pike
Rockville, MD 20852
(800) 638-8255

Information on aphasia and swallowing disorders. Referral to speech-language pathologists in your area.

Arthritis Foundation
P.O. Box 19000
Atlanta, GA 30326
(800) 283-7800

Offers the *Guide to Independent Living for People with Arthritis,* which is a 420-page manual that gives tips and illustrates and describes more than six hundred useful products for making daily activities easier. To order, send check for $11.95 ($9.95 plus $2.00 for shipping and handling).

Bible Alliance, Inc.
P. O. Box 621
Bradenton, FL 34206
(813) 748-3031

Free service for those who cannot read conventional print because of a visual or physical disability or visual impairment that prevents handling the printed material. The Bible on cassette, available in thirty-five languages, is given free of cost or obligation with proper verification of the impairment.

Children of Aging Parents (CAPS)
1609 Woodbourne Road, Suite 302-A
Levittown, PA 19057
(215) 945-6900

A national clearinghouse for caregivers of the elderly and professionals in the field of aging. Offers information and referral, publications on caregiving issues, and support groups.

Chrysler Corporation
Physically-Challenged Assistance Program
1220 Rankin Street
Troy, MI 48083-6004
(800) 255-9877

Offers (a) cash reimbursement to assist in reducing the cost of adaptive driving or passenger aids on new-model Chrysler cars, trucks, or vans; and (b) a resource center for information on adaptive products available to the physically challenged (free brochures).

The Dole Foundation
1819 H Street N.W., Suite 340
Washington, DC 20006-3603
(202) 457-0318
(202) 659-5315-TDD

Publishes *Workplace Workbook: Illustrated Guide to Job Accommodations and Assistive Technology*, to assist employers in making accommodations for workers with disabilities ($32.00). Order through the National Easter Seal Society, Publications Department, 70 East Lake Street, Chicago, IL 60601. Organizations seeking information about Dole Foundation grants should contact the foundation directly.

Epilepsy Foundation of America (EFA)
4351 Garden City Drive
Landover, MD 20785
(301) 459-3700
(800) 332-1000 (information/referral only)
(800) 332-4050 National Epilepsy Library (for professionals)

Family Caregiver Alliance
425 Bush Street, Suite 500
San Francisco, CA 94108
(415) 434-3388
(800) 445-8106 (in California)

Family support services for brain-impaired adults. Information and referral, fact sheets, and printed materials available nationwide. Service program for California residents only.

Federation of Special Care Organizations in Dentistry
211 East Chicago Avenue, Suite 1616
Chicago, IL 60611
(312) 440-2661

The federation includes the Association of Hospital Dentists, the Academy of Dentistry for the Handicapped, and the American Society for Geriatric Dentistry. It joins with organizations to continue improving the provision of quality oral health care, principally to the medically compromised, disabled, elderly, and frail who require special care.

Gerontological Society of America
1275 K Street, N.W., Suite 350
Washington, DC 20005-4006
(202) 842-1275

Expert referral service for professionals in the field of gerontology.

Gray Panthers
2025 Pennsylvania Avenue, N.W.
Washington, DC 20006
(202) 466-3132

Help for Incontinent People, Inc.
P. O. Box 544
Union, SC 29379
(803) 579-7900
(800) BLADDER (800 252-3337)

Help for Incontinent People (HIP) is a not-for-profit organization dedicated to improving the quality of life of people with incontinence. HIP is a leading source of education, advocacy, and support to the public and to the health profession about the causes, prevention, diagnosis, treatment of, and management alternatives for incontinence.

National Aphasia Association
Murray Hill Station
P. O. Box 1887
New York, NY 10156-0611
(800) 922-4NAA (800 922-4622)

Information about aphasia—reading list, fact sheet, newsletter, community groups, and volunteer regional representatives.

National Association of Area Agencies on Aging (NAAA)
1112-16th Street, N.W.
Suite 100
Washington, DC 20036
(202) 296-8130

A private, nonprofit organization representing the interests of Area Agencies on Aging (AAAs) across the country. Provides advocacy, legislative information, training, and technical assistance related to the management of AAAs and programs for the elderly, as well as provides consulting services to employers in the development and implementation of elder-care information and referral.

National Association for Hispanic Elderly
(Formerly National Association for Spanish-Speaking Elderly)
2025 I Street, N.W., Suite 219
Washington, DC 20006
(202) 293-9329

National Association for Music Therapy
8455 Colesville Road, Suite 930
Silver Spring, MD 20910
(301) 589-3300

Information and printed materials on use of music therapy.
Referral to music therapists in your area.

National Association of Professional Geriatric Care
Managers
655 North Alvernon Way, Suite 108
Tucson, AZ 85711
(602) 881-8008

An organization of practitioners whose goal is the advance-
ment of gentle and dignified care for the elderly and their
families.

National Association for Sickle Cell Disease, Inc.
3345 Wilshire Boulevard, Suite 1106
Los Angeles, CA 90010-1880
(213) 736-5455

A national organization providing research support, screening,
genetic counseling, vocational rehabilitation, scholarships,
and psychosocial and tutorial services. Seventy chapters.

National Center for Youth with Disabilities (NCYD)
University of Minnesota
Box 7214
20 Delaware Street, S.E.
Minneapolis, MN 55455
(800) 333-6293
(612) 626-2825
(612) 624-3939-TDD

An information and resource center focused on adolescents with chronic illnesses and disabilities and their transition to adult life. NCYD maintains a computerized database of current information and has a number of publications available.

National Council on the Aging, Inc.
409 Third Street, S.W., Suite 200
Washington, DC 20024
(202) 479-1200

National Council on Disability
1331 F Street, N.W., 10th Floor
Washington, DC 20004
(202) 267-3846 Voice
(202) 267-3232—TDD

An independent federal agency providing leadership in the identification of emerging issues and in the development and recommendation of disability policy that will promote equal opportunity and full integration of people with disabilities in society.

National Diabetes International Clearinghouse
Box NDIC
9000 Rockville Pike
Rockville, MD 20892
(301) 654-3327

Centralized resource for information on diabetes; consumer and professional publications, newsletter, and fact sheets.

National Digestive Diseases Information Clearinghouse
Box NDDIC
9000 Rockville Pike
Bethesda, MD 20892
(301) 654-3810

Provides information on products and services about digestive
diseases and disorders.

National Easter Seal Society
70 East Lake Street
Chicago, IL 60601
(312) 726-6200

Dedicated to increasing the independence of people with disabilities, adults and children. Information and printed materials available.

National Family Caregivers Association (NFCA)
9223 Longbranch Parkway
Silver Spring, MD 20901-3642
(301) 949-3638

A nonprofit membership organization serving family caregivers. Publishes a quarterly newsletter, *Take Care!*, which focuses on issues from the caregiver's perspective, and also runs
a speakers bureau. Membership is open to family caregivers,
professionals, and organizations.

National Handicapped Sports
451 Hungerford Drive, Suite 100
Rockville, MD 20850
(800) 966-4NHS (800-966-4647)

Promises sports and recreational activities nationwide for people with physical disabilities. Adaptive fitness and ski videos for sale.

National Information Center for Children and Youths with Disabilities (NICHCY)
P. O. Box 1492
Washington, DC 20013
(703) 893-6061
(800) 999-5599
(703) 893-8614—TDD

Provides free information to assist parents, educators, caregivers, advocates, and others in helping children and youth with disabilities to become participating members of the community. National clearinghouse; publications on current issues. Free brochures and fact sheets.

National Institute on Aging Information Center
P.O. Box 8057
Gaithersburg, MD 20898-8057
(800) 222-2225 - Voice
(800) 222-4225-TDD

Publications clearinghouse providing free materials to all persons interested in healthful aging. Available information includes fact sheets, pamphlets, and technical reports on disease prevention, health education, aging research, medical care, nutrition, safety, the body, and more.

National Institute on Aging (NIA) Public Information Office
Building 31, Room 5C27
9000 Rockville Pike
Bethesda, MD 20892
(301) 496-1752

Responsible for the conduct and support of biomedical, social, and behavioral research; training; health-information dissemination; and other programs with respect to the aging process and the diseases and other special problems and needs of the aged.

National Kidney and Urologic Diseases Information
Clearinghouse
Box NKUDIC
9000 Rockville Pike
Bethesda, MD 20892
(301) 468-8345

Clearinghouse providing information and referrals about products and services related to kidney and urologic diseases.

National Library Service for the Blind and Physically
Handicapped
Library of Congress
1291 Taylor Street, N.W.
Washington, DC 20542
(800) 424-9100

Provides Braille and recorded books and magazines, catalogs and bibliographies, music scores, and music-instruction material free for blind and physically handicapped persons. Talking-book players and accessories necessary in order to use the cassettes and records are also provided without cost.

National Rehabilitation Association
1910 Association Drive, Suite 205
Reston, VA 22091-1502
(703) 715-9090

National Rehabilitation Information Center (NARIC) and
ABLEDATA
8455 Colesville Road, Suite 935
Silver Spring, MD 20910-3319
(800) 227-0216 - Voice/TDD
(301) 588-9284 - Voice/TDD

Computer database for information on rehabilitation and
health-related problems. Publications and materials available.

National Self-Help Clearinghouse
Graduate School and University Center of the City
University of New York
25 West 43rd Street, Room 620
New York, NY 10036
(212) 642-2944

Information and referral for location of self-help groups.
Conducts training activities; publishes manual and a newsletter.

North American Riding for the Handicapped, Inc.
P. O. Box 33150
Denver, CO 80233
(800) 369-RIDE (800-369-7433)
(303) 452-1212

Promotes the recovery of individuals with disabilities through
therapeutic horseback riding. Call for a list of member centers
in your state.

Parent Care
Gerontology Center
4089 Dole Building
Human Development Center
University of Kansas
Lawrence, KS 66045
(913) 864-4130

Resources to assist family caregivers.

The President's Committee on Employment of People with
Disabilities
1331 F Street, N.W.
Washington, DC 20004-1107
(202) 376-6200 (Voice)
(202) 376-6205 (TDD)

A federal agency that enhances the employment of people
with disabilities. Provides information, training, and technical
assistance to America's business leaders, rehabilitation and
service providers, advocacy organizations, families and individuals with disabilities, and supervises the Job Accommoda-
tion Network (JAN), a free service that provides information
and consulting on accommodating persons with disabilities in
the workplace. This service may be accessed by phone—(800)
526-7234—or by computer bulletin board—(800) 342-5526.

Rehabilitation Research and Training Center for Brain
Injury and Stroke
University of Washington
Department of Rehabilitation
Medicine RJ-30
Seattle, WA 98195

Write for information.

The Simon Foundation for Continence
P. O. Box 815
Wilmette, IL 6009
(708) 864-3913
(800) 237-4666 (patient information)

Dedicated to helping people with incontinence—the loss of
bowel and/or bladder control. Provides books, tapes, newsletters, and reprints. Also sponsors "I Will Manage" educational
support groups.

United Seniors Health Cooperative
1331 H Street, N.W., #500
Washington, DC 20005-4706
(202) 393-6222

United Seniors Health Cooperative (USHC) is a not-for-profit
organization dedicated to improving the quality of life and
reducing the cost of health and social services for older adults.
USHC has published several highly acclaimed books, conducted numerous health insurance studies, and publishes a
newsletter for older consumers.

United Way of America
701 North Fairfax Street
Alexandria, VA 22314-2045
(703) 836-7100

Very Special Arts USA
Education Office
The John F. Kennedy Center for Performing Arts Center
Washington, DC 20056
(800) 933-8721
(202) 737-0645 TDD

International opportunities in music, dance, drama, literature, and visual arts to individuals with mental and physical challenges. Organizations in each state.

Veterans Administration (VA)
810 Vermont Avenue, N.W.
Washington, DC 20420
(202) 233-4000

Visiting Nurse Associations of America
3801 East Florida Avenue, Suite 206
Denver, CO 80210
(800) 426-2547

Information and referrals for home health care services—PT, OT, speech, general nursing. More than four hundred locations nationwide. Free brochure.

Wayne State University Press
The Leonard N. Simons Building
5959 Woodward Avenue
Detroit, MI 48202
(313) 577-6120

Publications and videos on speech and language pathology. For information and free brochures, contact Mike Ware.

The Well Spouse Foundation
P.O. Box 801
New York, NY 10023
(212) 724-7209 (9:00 A.M.–9:00 P.M. eastern time)

A nationwide organization that provides support for the husbands, wives, and partners of the chronically ill. Bimonthly newsletter, regional support groups, pen-pal system, advocacy program.

RESOURCES FOR HOME AND VEHICLE EQUIPMENT

American Medical Industries
330½ East Third Street
Dell Rapids, SD 57022
(605) 428-5501
(605) 428-5502 fax

Carries EZ-SWALLOW Pill Crushers and Splitters, which crush medications into a fine powder or cut them into equal portions with a twist of the wrist or snap of the cap. Also available are the *Mayo Clinic Heart Book* and Electronic Pill Box with Timer.

Aquatec Health Care Products, L.P.
P.I.I.P.-I.C.M. Building
1003 International Drive
Oakdale, PA 15071-9223
(412) 695-2122
(412) 695-2922 fax

Aquatec Bathlifts provide safe transportation into and out of the bathtub. They're powered by water pressure, easy to install, and usually require no changes in the original plumbing. Two-year warranty. Free brochures.

Barrier Free Lifts, Inc.
P.O. Box 4163
Manassas, VA 22110
(800) 582-8732 or (703) 361-6531
(703) 361-7861 fax

Barrier Free Ceiling Lifts are available in many models for lifting and moving people. The "Portable" model can be transferred between different tracks. Other lifts range from manual to fully motorized. Optional controls include nonelectric air tubes and wireless-radio-controlled. Battery operated and easy to use, they lift, lower, and move along a track.

The Braun Corporation
P. O. Box 310
Winamac, Indiana 46996
(800) THE-LIFT

Supplies van lifts, including Entervan, The Tri-Wheeler, and Chair Topper.

Bruce Medical Supply
411 Waverly Oaks Road
P. O. Box 9166
Waltham, MA 02254
(800) 225-8446

This mail-order medical supplier may save you up to 60 percent on home health care needs. They carry a complete selection of dressing, grooming, dining, and mobility aids; incontinent, bedroom, and bathroom items; diabetic, ostomy, laryngectomy, and tracheostomy supplies; and nutritious foods. 100 percent satisfaction guarantee. Orders are shipped the day they are received.

Bruno Independent Living Aids, Inc.
P. O. Box 841780
Executive Drive
Oconomowoc, WI 53066
(800) 882-8183 or (414) 567-4990
(414) 567-4341 fax

Bruno Electra-Ride is a low-cost, battery-powered stairway elevator that requires no special wiring. Capacity rated to 350 pounds. Includes retractable seatbelt, two remote call-sends, contoured seating, full swivel top and bottom, adjustable footplate, and soft-start controller with dependable rack-and-pinion drive.

Bruno Regal Scooter Series: Three- and four-wheel RWD and FWD scooters, including the Regal Pediatric. RWD with slant platform, proportional sizing, contoured seating, E-Z Tilt tiller, 1.32-hp motor and take-apart construction. Can be used indoors and outdoors.

Bruno Scooter-Lift Jr.: One of fourteen different lifts available to eliminate the burden of transporting wheelchairs and scooters. Bruno Lifts can be installed in nearly any car, van, mini-van or truck, both foreign and domestic, for full or partially assembled mobility aids. Free brochures.

Collis Curve
313 West 48th Street
Minneapolis, MN 55409
(612) 822-2740
(612) 822-7209 fax

Collis Curve Toothbrush has curved bristles that remove plaque and massage the gums, making brushing easy and efficient for everyone, especially the disabled. Only toothbrush with A.D.A. Seal for Assisted Brushing Technique.

Damaco Freedom on Wheels
20542 Plummer Street
Chatsworth, CA 91311
(800) 432-2434 or (818) 709-4534
(818) 709-5282 fax

Portable, lightweight power and manual wheelchairs in custom sizes for youngsters and adults. The Applause "Super-Hemi" height ranges from 14½ to 17½ inches. Damaco's D90 Power Conversion System converts most manual wheelchairs to power. Free catalog.

Greatest of Ease Company
2443 Fillmore, #345
San Francisco, CA 94115
(800) 845-1208
(415) 441-4319 fax

Call help from more than one hundred feet away without shouting and phone call. Battery-operated, wireless Personal Pager fits into pocket or purse. Press transmitter button and pager beeps; works through most walls. Can also be used outdoors. $39.95 plus $4.00 shipping. Ten-day money-back guarantee.

Homecare Products, Inc.
15824 S.E. 296th Street
Kent, WA 98042
(800) 451-1903
(206) 630-8196 fax

Manufacturers of EZ-Access portable wheelchair ramps. Available in three-, five-, seven-, eight-, and ten-foot lengths. EZ-Access Ramps can be found at dealers and distributors nationwide. Free brochures.

Jesana, Ltd.
P.O. Box 17
Irvington, NY 10533
(800) 443-4728

A full-service mail-order catalog offering a full spectrum of devices for the physically disabled. Free catalogs.

Knobbles
7235 South Steele Circle
Department SA
Littleton, CO 80122-1940
(800) 346-5662

Knobbles are soft, ribbed thermoplastic sleeves that slip over existing doorknobs, making doorknobs easier to grip and turn for weak hands. Knobbles are available in brown, bronze, and glow-in-the-dark colors and cost $5.00 for four.

Lumex, Division of Lumex, Inc.
81 Spence Street
Bay Shore, NY 11706
(516) 273-2200
(516) 273-5681 fax

Lumex is a leading manufacturer of health care equipment for home and institutional use. The company's product lines include bathroom-safety products, walking aids, specialty seating, bathing systems, wheelchairs, therapeutic support systems, and other patient-care equipment. Free catalog.

Merry Walker Corporation
1357 Northmoore Court
Northbrook, IL 60062
(708) 498-9028
(708) 498-5920 fax

The new Walk Master is a new ambulation device developed by the inventor of the original Merry Walker. It allows the user to be completely restraint-free and walk independently, helping to restore healthy functioning of ambulatory status, respiration, and circulation. Approved for Medicare reimbursement. Free brochure.

Rifton for People with Disabilities
P.O. Box 901
Rifton, NY 12471-0901
(800) 374-3866
(914) 658-8065 Fax

This company provides lift walkers, mobile standers, walkers, chairs, and standers for the adult in need of assistance. Free catalog.

Smith & Nephew Rolyan
One Quality Drive
P.O. Box 578
Germantown, WI 53022
(800) 558-8633
(800) 545-7758 fax

Free catalog contains a selection of high-quality assistive devices that enable people to improve daily-living activities. Included are homemaking, eating, dressing, grooming, and writing aids.

Stow Away, Inc.
513 South Pine Street
Chelsea, OK 74016
(800) 221-3433

Light, strong, and competitively priced power-operated wheelchair and scooter lifts, including a Fly & Drive model.

Simple installation, easy to transfer between vehicles. One-year warranty. Free brochures.

Texim International
17777 Main Street, Suite H
Irvine, CA 92714
(800) 942-4249
(714) 261-9125 fax

Texima Magnetic Latch replaces interior-door passage sets. Holds door closed by magnetic force and eliminates turning of the knob or lever. The magnetic force of the latch is adjustable to meet the requirements of the user. Privacy can be added with Texima Mortise Bolt. Free catalog.

TFH (USA), Ltd.
4449 Gibsonia Road
Gibsonia, PA 15044
(412) 444-6400

TFH (USA) has two catalogs: "Age Appropriate Resources," which includes games, amusements, and recreation for teens to geriatrics; and "Fun and Achievement," which includes adapted products and toys for children to teens.

RESOURCES FOR CLOTHING AND DRESSING AIDS

Bruce Medical Supply
411 Waverly Oaks Road
P. O. Box 9166
Waltham, MA 02254
(800) 225-8446

Mail-order medical supplier saves you up to 60 percent on your home health care needs. Complete selection of dressing and grooming aids, as well as other home health care equipment. 100 percent satisfaction guarantee. Orders are shipped the day they are received.

Buck and Buck Clothing
3111 27th Avenue South
Seattle, WA 98144
(206) 722-4196
(206) 722-1144 fax

Clothing and accessories for nursing-home residents. A full line of regular washable clothing, as well as clothing for special needs, for men and women. Shoes, wheelchair accessories, and room accessories. Free catalog.

D. Greene & Associates
5502 Kenilworth Avenue, Suite 305
Riverdale, MD 20737
(800) 448-7079

Depends adult briefs, bed pads, and liners are available by the case at low prices and delivered to the patient's home. Other personal-care products are also available. Free catalog.

Hen's Nest
P. O. Box 531
Colby, KS 67701
(913) 426-3104

Custom-made clothing for children and adults. Basic designs available. Free brochures.

Laborie Medical Technologies Corp.
7 Green Tree Drive
South Burlington, VT 05403
(800) 522-3393
(802) 860-1147 fax

Active Living Catalog contains absorbent products, reusables, catheters, and accessories for the management of urinary incontinence. All products are shipped to the home in unmarked boxes. Free catalog.

Maddak Inc.
6 Industrial Road
Pequannock, NJ 07440
(201) 628-7600

Maddak Inc. is a manufacturer and supplier of ADLs and rehabilitative devices. A complete selection of dressing, grooming, bed, and bathroom aids is available. Free catalog.

M. J. Markell Shoe Company, Inc.
504 Saw Mill River Road
Yonkers, NY 10702
(914) 963-2258
(914) 963-9293 fax

Markell offers a variety of stock accommodative footwear for adults, such as the washable Pulman International comfort shoes. Special stock, extra-deep mobility shoes for diabetics and arthritics are also available. Shoes are in stock and available nationwide through shoe stores and orthotic and prosthetic facilities.

Maxi-Aids
P.O. Box 3209
Farmingdale, NY 11735
(800) 522-6294
(516) 752-0689 fax

Products for the visually impaired, hearing impaired, arthritic, and physically challenged: magnifiers, low-vision books, games, eating and dressing aids, radios, listening systems, bathroom aids, kitchen appliances, and more. Free catalog.

Priva, Inc.
P.O. Box 448
Champlain, NY 12919-0448
(800) 361-4964
(514) 356-0055 fax

Reusable incontinence care products are available from this company: bed and chair pads, briefs for heavy-to-light incontinence, liners, and washable bibs.

Smith & Nephew Rolyan
One Quality Drive
P.O. Box 578
Germantown, WI 53022
(800) 558-8633
(800) 545-7758 fax

Free catalog contains a selection of assistive devices that enable people to improve their daily-living activities. Included are homemaking, eating, dressing, grooming, and writing aids.

RESOURCES FOR RECREATION, TRAVEL, AND EXERCISE

Access to Recreation, Inc.
2509 East Thousand Oaks Boulevard, Suite 430
Thousand Oaks, CA 91362
(800) 634-4351 or (805) 498-7535
(805) 498-8186 fax

Adapted equipment for exercise, fishing, bowling, skiing, and other activities for the physically challenged. Lifts for access to swimming pool, wheelchairs, and grasping gloves, ramps, books, and other items, including aids for daily living, are also available. Money-back guarantee. Free catalog.

Access Tours, Inc.
Box 2985
Jackson, WY 83001
(800) 929-4811

Package tours of Yellowstone, Glacier Park, Grand Canyon, Bryce Canyon, Zion, southern Arizona, and other special areas are available to individuals or groups. Trips are accessible for mobility-impaired persons with wheelchair-lift-equipped vehicles.

Adaptability
Department 2228
Colchester, CT 06415
(800) 288-9941
(800) 566-6678 fax

Products for independent living: mobility aids, therapy, ADL, exercise, kitchen and home aids, evaluation, rehabilitation. Free catalog.

Bruce Medical Supply
411 Waverly Oaks Road
P.O. Box 9166
Waltham, MA 02254
(800) 225-8446

Complete selection of mobility aids and health care equipment. 100 percent satisfaction guarantee. Orders are shipped the day they are received. Free catalog.

Senior Fitnessize
P.O. Box 2567
Morganton, NC 28655
(704) 438-9274

Audiotape and/or manual with videotape to assist with range-of-motion and muscle-toning exercises. All exercises are performed while seated. Free catalog.

TFH (USA), Ltd.
4449 Gibsonia Road
Gibsonia, PA 15044
(412) 444-6400

TFH (USA) has two catalogs: "Age Appropriate Resources," which includes games, amusements, and recreation for teens to geriatrics; and "Fun and Achievement," which includes adapted products and toys for children to teens.

Travelin' Talk
P.O. Box 3534
Clarksville, TN 37043
(615) 552-6670

Membership network of people assisting travelers with disabilities; quarterly newsletter with news, tips, resources; five-hundred-page directory of resources. Membership: onetime registration fee on sliding scale. Newsletter available for contribution. Directory and catalog, $35.00 each.

RESOURCES FOR COMMUNICATION AND COMPUTERS

Attainment Company, Inc.
P.O. Box 930160
Verona, WI 53593-0160
(800) 327-4269
(800) 942-3865 fax

Attainment Company has two affordable Pocket Talkers for receptive and expressive communication. Each Pocket Talker records and plays five different messages using digital recording. Free catalog.

Bruce Medical Supply
411 Waverly Oaks Road
P. O. Box 9166
Waltham, MA 02254
(800) 225-8446

Complete selection of communication devices and other health care equipment. 100 percent satisfaction guarantee. Orders are shipped the day they are received. Free catalog.

Crestwood Company
6625 North Sidney Place
Milwaukee, WI 53209
(414) 352-5678
(414) 352-5679 fax

This company offers three hundred types of devices, including Talking Pictures and communication boards, Opticommunicator Maxx for paralyzed people to "talk with their eyes," light and high-tech switches and aids, and a large selection of adapted and voice-activated toys. Free catalog.

Greatest of Ease Company
2443 Fillmore, #345
San Francisco, CA 94115
(800) 845-1208
(415) 441-4319 fax

Call help from more than one hundred feet away without shouting and phone call. Battery-operated, wireless Personal Pager fits into pocket or purse. Press transmitter button and pager beeps; works through most walls. Can also use outdoors. $39.95 plus $4.00 shipping. Ten-day money-back guarantee.

Hearing Resources
5215 Southeast 52nd Avenue
Portland, OR 97206
(503) 774-3668
(503) 774-7247 fax

This company supplies such items as flashing signals for doorbell, telephone, clock, emergency paging, and home security. Amplifying systems for a variety of listening situations are also available, including television, telephone, talking in cars, within small groups in restaurants, business meetings, theaters, and churches. Vibrating timers for pill taking also available. Free catalog.

IBM National Support Center for Persons with Disabilities
1000 Northwest 51st Street
Boca Raton, FL 33432
(800) 426-4832 (Voice)
(800) 465-7999 (Canada)
(800) 426-4833 (TDD)
(407) 982-6059 fax

This company provides information on how computers can help people with vision, hearing, speech, learning, mental-retardation, and mobility problems. Assistive devices and software are available. Free product fact sheets.

Imaginart Communication Products
307 Arizona Street
Bisbee, AZ 85603
(602) 432-5741 or (800) 828-1376
(602) 432-5134 fax

This company provides a variety of devices, including the Pick'n Stick sticker system for augmentative communication. Speech and language materials for children and adults, including photo cards, workbooks, Word-Finding Program, Thick-it, and swallowing and aphasia materials are also available. Free catalog.

Interactive Therapeutics, Inc.
P.O. Box 1805
Stow, OH 44224-0805
(216) 688-1371 or (800) 253-5111
(216) 688-1055 fax

Printed word "Daily Communicator" and "Picture Communicator" notebooks in two sizes—pocket sized ($3\frac{1}{2}'' \times 6''$) and enlarged ($5'' \times 8^{1}/_{2}''$)—are available from this company. Educational counseling booklets on aphasia, dysarthria, apraxia, and head injury, and the "Let's Organize Today" daily planner with more than four hundred activities to help facilitate communication and thinking skills are among the materials available for adolescent and adult rehabilitation. Free catalog.

Microsystems Software, Inc.
600 Worcester Road
Framingham, MA 01701
(800) 828-2600
(508) 626-8515 fax

HandiWARE and MAGIC, special-needs software solutions for individuals with mobility, speech and hearing impairment, and low vision are among the products available from this company. Provides screen magnification and adapted access to any DOS or Windows application by assisting individuals with limited keyboarding ability, severe physical involvement, speech impairment, or no speech. Free catalog.

Prentke Romich Company
1022 Heyl Road
Wooster, OH 44691
(800) 262-1984
(216) 263-4829 fax

This company is the largest manufacturer of augmentative- and alternative-communication systems providing interactive communication for nonspeaking people. The company also manufactures and distributes computer products for speech- and mobility-impaired individuals. Free catalog.

Thought Technology
c/o Cimetra
8396 Route 9 North
West Chazy, NY 12992
(800) 361-3651 or (514) 489-8251
(514) 489-8255 fax

This leading manufacturer of biofeedback equipment for muscle reeducation provides portable home trainers and computer-based clinical instrumentation to assist with dysphasia and muscle strengthening. Equipment scans to detect residual muscle activity, then provides visual and tonal feedback to help in retraining.

Tolfa Corporation
1001 North Rengstorff Avenue
Mountain View, CA 94043
(800) 332-4913

Supplies Lingraphica, an FDA-regulated, clinically proven language prosthesis for aphasia. It is an integrated system that combines spoken words, printed words, images, and text processing to make full use of a person's communicative abilities. Free brochure.

RESOURCES FOR BOOKS, VIDEOTAPES, AUDIOTAPES, AND FILMS

American Source Books
Department 179
P.O. Box 1094
San Luis Obispo, CA 93406
(805) 543-5911

Publishes resource books for caregivers. Recent titles include *Keeping Active: A Caregiver's Guide to Activities with the Elderly, Long Distance Caregiving,* and *Hiring Home Helpers.* Also publishes *Caring Ways,* a free newsletter full of time-saving, money-saving, stress-reducing tips for caregivers. Free catalog.

A/V Health Services, Inc.
P.O. Box 20271
Roanoke, VA 24018
(703) 389-4339
(703) 389-4339 fax

Produces instructional and exercise videotapes for the physically challenged, with a special focus on activities of daily living. Free catalog.

Danamar Productions
106 Monte Vista Place
Santa Fe, NM 87501
(800) 578-6508

Provides *The Healing Influence: Guidelines for Stroke Families,* an award-winning video hosted by Patricia Neal. Endorsed by The American Heart Association and Heart/Stroke Foundation of Canada. "Ms. Neal's presentation is not only a prescription for recovery, it's a triumphant inspiration to others." Special stroke-club price: $44.95; institutional price: $299.00.

Harmarville Rehabilitation Center
P.O. Box 11460
Guys Run Road
Pittsburgh, PA 15238
(800) 624-HOPE (800-624-4673)

The center offers *Road to Access,* video instructions for physically challenged travelers and their companions on methods and techniques for traveling by air, train, bus, and subway. Cost: $19.95.

Occu-Ther, Inc.
11316 Lakeshore Drive West
Carmel, IN 46033

Provides a video exercise program for the stroke survivor emphasizing the use of one's strong side to mobilize the weak side. Designed and developed by an occupational therapist. Performed in the sitting position. Free catalog.

OTHER SERVICES

Athena Rx Home Pharmacy
800 Q Gateway Boulevard
South San Francisco, CA 94080
(800) 528-4362
(415) 877-8370 fax

Savings on chronic maintenance medications and access to important support services (*Neurology Awareness* newsletter, free express air-courier delivery, refill reminders, aid with insurance, private pharmacy consultations, and more). Call 9:00 A.M.–9:00 P.M. EST, or twenty-four hours in an emergency.

Enrichments
145 Tower Drive
Burr Ridge, IL 60521
(800) 323-5547

Offers adaptive items to simplify daily tasks: preparing and eating meals, reading a book, cleaning the home, buttoning a shirt, or zipping trousers. Easy-to-dress clothing with all-Velcro closures also available. Free catalog.

Harmarville Rehabilitation Center
P.O. Box 11460
Guys Run Road
Pittsburgh, PA 15238
(800) 624-HOPE (800-624-4673)

A two-hundred bed, nonprofit rehabilitation center providing inpatient and outpatient physical medicine and rehabilitation for adults. NSA chapter site.

The Hillhaven Corporation
1148 Broadway Plaza
Tacoma, WA 98402
(800) 526-5782 or (206) 572-4901

Stroke, cardiopulmonary conditions, orthopedics, multiple traumas, IV therapies, and cancer are a focus of this organization's Steps Ahead Subacute Medical and Rehabilitation Program. The corporation has more than three hundred locations nationwide and includes physiatrist-directed programs with internal case management, on-staff therapists, and specially trained twenty-four-hour R.N. staffing.

Menu Magic
1717 West 10th Street
Indianapolis, IN 46222
(800) 732-5805

Menu Magic is a manufacturer of specialty nutritional foods and liquid thickeners to assist those with swallowing problems. Products are available through Bruce Medical Supply and Med Diet, (800) MED DIET.

NovaCare, Inc.
1016 West Ninth Avenue
King of Prussia, PA 19406
(215) 992-7200
(800) 331-8840

NovaCare, Inc., is the largest provider of contract rehabilitation therapy and orthotic and prosthetic patient-care services in the United States. In addition the company operates twelve acute-care medical rehabilitation hospitals and a number of freestanding comprehensive outpatient rehabilitation facilities and community-reentry programs. With operations in forty-two states, NovaCare employees currently treat more than twenty-six thousand patients per day.

Spalding Rehabilitation Hospital
4500 East Iliff Avenue
Denver, CO 80222
(303) 782-5703

Comprehensive rehabilitation of patients with musculoskeletal problems, occupational injuries, and neurological disorders such as stroke, multiple sclerosis, and brain injury. Post-Stroke Clinic provides medical and functional evaluation of stroke survivors living in the community who have noticed changes in their ability to function physically, socially, or emotionally.

Glossary

accessibility Refers to the relative ease with which an obstacle (e.g., curb or ramp) can be negotiated or a facility or vehicle can be reached or entered by people using crutches or wheelchairs or who are otherwise restricted in mobility.

agnosia A perceptual impairment resulting in inability to recognize familiar objects or associate an object with its use (e.g., using toothbrush to comb hair).

aneurysm Small, blisterlike weak spots in the walls of blood vessels, which may rupture and cause hemorrhage (bleeding). Cause of a small percentage of strokes.

ankle-foot orthosis Brace used to support weak or paralyzed ankle and foot muscle in order to simulate normal joint movement, enhance walking ability, and prevent further injury.

aphasia Communication impairment resulting in inability to express oneself by speaking, writing, or gesturing (expressive aphasia) and/or inability to understand written or spoken language (receptive aphasia).

apraxia Speech disorder that makes it difficult to "program" speech in an understandable manner. Sounds are often made correctly, but in the wrong order. Also, a perceptual and cognitive impairment resulting in an inability to perform certain purposeful movements despite presence of adequate strength, sensation, and coordination; same movements may be done automatically at other times.

arm trough A device usually attached to the arm of a wheelchair for the purpose of supporting a flaccid or weak upper extremity.

arteriosclerosis Thickening or loss of elasticity in arterial walls. Also called hardening of the arteries.

aspiration Entry of any foreign substance (for example, food) below the level of the vocal cords.

ataxia Movement impairment from a brain lesion causing lack of coordination, unsteady gait, and poor balance.

atherosclerosis A condition caused by fatty deposits along the inner lining of blood vessels (especially arteries) resulting in narrowing of the vessel and restriction of blood flow.

atrial fibrillation A heart condition in which the heart beats in an irregular fashion. Atrial fibrillation is a stroke risk factor.

cane A walking aid, made of wood or metal, to be held in one hand for the purpose of enhancing balance and stability.

cardiovascular Refers to heart and blood vessels.

carotid artery Principal artery on either side of the neck, which carries blood from the heart to the brain.

catheter A rubber tube for collection of urine from a person with a disturbance of bladder function, as after a stroke.

diuretic Type of medication that washes out salt (sodium) from the body and helps to reduce high blood pressure and edema.

drop-foot A foot that dangles when the leg is lifted, because of weakness or paralysis of the ankle and foot muscles; can be alleviated with a brace.

dysarthria Impairment in articulation, resulting from weakness in mouth, tongue, and jaw, causing slurred speech.

dysphagia Impairment in swallowing.

edema Swelling of body parts due to excessive fluid in the tissue spaces.

embolism The sudden blocking of an artery or vein by a clot carried by the bloodstream from one part of the body to the point of obstruction; one cause of stroke.

esophagus Body's passageway from throat to stomach.

flaccidity Absence of muscle tone, resulting in a floppy, nonfunctional limb.

gait Manner of walking; normal gait cycle has a swing phase and a stance phase for each lower limb; gait training—specific therapeutic neuromuscular techniques used by a physical therapist on trunk and limbs combined with instructions to the patient for enhancing muscle responses for improved walking pattern.

grab bar A bar, usually metal, solidly fixed to a wall, as in a bathtub, to provide support for persons with balance or strength impairments.

hemianopsia Permanent damage to the optic nerve, which results in blindness in one-half of each eye. The same half of each eye is affected as the side of the body that is affected by stroke. Therapy or glasses will not change this vision problem, but compensation techniques can be learned.

hemiparesis Weakness on one side of the body; may include head and neck, trunk and limbs.

hemiplegia Paralysis, or loss of voluntary motion, on one side of the body; may include head and neck, trunk and limbs.

hemorrhage Bleeding; one cause of stroke if it occurs in the brain.

hypertension Abnormally high blood pressure; can lead to stroke or heart disease.

impairment A disturbance in an organ or system in the body due to an injury, disorder, or disease.

incontinence Involuntary discharge of urine or feces.

ischemia Lack of oxygen in localized area of body, as in part of the brain.

joint A junction between the ends of two or more bones in the skeleton, surrounded by muscles and other supportive tissue; joints allow for varying degrees of normal motion among the bones.

lability Impairment of emotional control after brain damage; usually manifests as frequent, brief episodes of spontaneous crying or laughing with no obvious stimulus; usually resolves during stroke recovery.

lapboard A board of wood or plastic secured across the arms of a wheelchair to provide both support for a hemiplegic upper limb and an eating and working surface.

neglect, one-sided Unconscious perceptual impairment resulting in lack of awareness of the side of the body and environment on the affected side; if combined with hemianopsia, there is high potential for injury.

neurologist Physician specializing in the brain and nervous system who usually treats people with acute stroke until their transfer to a rehabilitation setting.

neuromuscular Refers to the interaction of the brain and nervous system with the muscular and skeletal systems to produce movement.

occupational therapy (OT) Rehabilitation specialty that assists disabled persons to regain fulfilling daily occupations of leisure and work through training in perceptual and cognitive skills and daily activities, leading to improved self-esteem and quality of life.

orthosis An external device applied to a part of the body for a supportive, adaptive, preventive, or corrective purpose; includes braces, splints, and other devices.

paralysis Loss or impairment of voluntary movement by a muscle or groups of muscles due to injury or disease of the neuromuscular system.

perception The ability to receive, interpret, and use information through the sensory systems (vision, touch, taste, etc.).

physiatrist Physician specializing in physical medicine; member of rehabilitation team who cares for medical problems during rehabilitation.

physical therapy (PT) Rehabilitation specialty concerned with helping those with impairments from disease, injury, or surgery to prevent disability and pain, restore functional movement and ambulations, promote healing, and adapt to permanent disabilities.

pocketing Refers to the habit of getting food caught between the cheek and gum on the paralyzed side of the face; results in food not being chewed, swallowed, or digested properly.

positioning Helping a stroke survivor position himself or herself in bed, on a chair, or elsewhere in a position that offsets spastic patterns, allows functional activity, and otherwise minimizes the dangers of faulty posture, such as contractures, pressure sores, impaired breathing; may require use of pillows, splints, or other supports.

pressure sore Skin breakdown resulting from prolonged pressure on one spot, usually from sitting or lying in one position too long; also called bedsore or decubitus ulcer.

range of motion (ROM) The extent of available (passive) movement in a particular joint; can be affected by disease, injury, or muscle stiffness; relates to both the ROM test a therapist does and to the ROM exercises taught for the purpose of maintaining or increasing joint motion and muscle flexibility.

recreational therapy (RT) The use of recreational or leisure-time activities as a therapeutic part of the rehabilitation process; a specialized field of knowledge practiced by certified RTs.

rehabilitation The restoration of an individual, after a disabling disease, injury, or condition, to the maximum of his or her physical, mental, social, spiritual, and vocational potentials; ideally done by the individual in team with rehabilitation professionals.

relaxation exercises Techniques of systematic attention to muscle tone, posture, and breathing for the purpose of relaxing the body and mind.

skilled-nursing facility/care A long-term institutional setting where continuous nursing and medical care are provided; for people with chronic medical problems who need a moderate to maximal amount of assistance; some rehabilitation therapies may be available.

sliding board A smooth wood or plastic board about two feet long used for transfers of people unable to stand on at least one lower limb. Also called a transfer board.

sling Soft support, usually of canvas, for a body part; after stroke, often needed to support a weakened shoulder.

spasm A sudden, involuntary contraction of a muscle or group of muscles with pain and disturbance of function; as differentiated from spasticity.

spasticity A state of increase over normal tension (tone) of a muscle, resulting in continuous resistance to stretching.

speech pathology The study and treatment of disorders in the field of human communication, including speech and language, writing, reading; also referred to as speech therapy.

splint A type of orthosis; usually small, light, one-piece, fitted to support a body part in a desired position, such as a resting-hand splint after a stroke.

stroke Sudden loss of function of a part of the brain due to interference in its blood supply, usually by thrombosis or hemorrhage.

stroke club A community group organized to provide emotional support and social activities for stroke survivors and their families; often initiated and run by the participants rather than a professional.

stroke support group Small groups of people who are not stroke survivors themselves, but may be caregivers or otherwise involved with stroke survivors; its purpose is to provide support and an opportunity for resolving personal concerns; usually coordinated by a counselor or rehabilitation professional.

thrombosis The formation, development, or presence of a blood clot in a blood vessel; cause of stroke if in blood vessels leading to or in the brain.

transfers Movement from one position to another; usually from one seat to another, such as from bed to chair, wheelchair to car, and so forth.

transient ischemic attack (TIA) A brief or temporary episode of neurological symptoms (such as blurred vision, slurred speech, numbness, weakness, or loss of balance), which may disappear but may be a forewarning of a stroke; also called ministroke.

vascular Pertaining to the blood supply or to blood tissues.

Velcro Material that can be glued or sewn onto clothing to replace zippers and buttons; has two layers, which adhere to each other; can be easily manipulated with one hand.

work-capacity evaluation Recently-developed science of analyzing the precise physical and mental task demands involved in jobs so as to match them more carefully to the specific skills and capacities of a disabled person.

Index